Praise for *The Mindful Path to Intimacy*

"Dr. Cordova provides heartfelt guidance for the challenges of honoring ourselves and another in meaningful, intertwined lives. The useful exercises and examples throughout the book will deepen your learning. I highly recommend this book for any couple, whether you are struggling or not. There is wisdom for all of us here."

—Lizabeth Roemer, PhD,
Department of Psychology,
University of Massachusetts Boston

"This book came into my life at just the right time. Being guided with actionable scripts and the tools to find solutions has made me feel immensely supported. I was surprised to discover that, with vulnerability and a bit of humor, simply identifying our relationship patterns (mountains and molehills here) eases friction in moments of conflict, and is helping me and my partner find deeper trust and connection."

—Dominique H., Denver

"I cherish the skills I am learning from this book. Dr. Cordova provides tangible tools to nurture intimate relationships."

—Jessica S., Albuquerque

"Dr. Cordova is a skilled therapist with a particular gift for imagery that gets to the heart of common relationship struggles. This book invites couples to turn toward each other for comfort and closeness, even when stress or hurt feelings get in the way. Dr. Cordova outlines mindfulness practices that can help you create a deeper, richer, more resilient relationship."

—Kristina Coop Gordon, PhD,
coauthor of *Getting Past the Affair, Second Edition*

"From being mindful of our daily actions and listening deeply to each other, to understanding our differing styles of attachment, it's hard to imagine ever floundering in our relationship again when these meaningful words and pointed guidance are sitting on our bookshelf."

—Nicole D., Worcester, Massachusetts

"Dr. Cordova's profound insights and practical strategies are helping me and my partner deepen our relationship further, even though we have been together for decades."

—Van C., Denver

"Dr. Cordova borrows from attachment theory and the ancient practice of mindfulness meditation to provide a new look at couple relationships. He describes how intimacy can be damaged in the rough and tumble of our daily lives, and shows a path toward repairing it. I firmly believe that following the strategies in this book with your partner can help you experience greater connection."

—Andrew Christensen, PhD,
coauthor of *Reconcilable Differences, Second Edition*

THE MINDFUL PATH TO INTIMACY

The Mindful Path to Intimacy

CULTIVATING A DEEPER CONNECTION WITH YOUR PARTNER

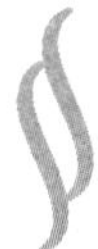

James V. Cordova, PhD

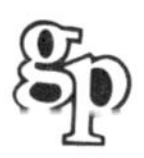

THE GUILFORD PRESS
New York London

A Division of Guilford Publications, Inc.
www.guilford.com

The information in this volume is not intended as a substitute for consultation with health care professionals. Each individual's health concerns should be evaluated by a qualified professional.

Printed in the United States of America

Last digit is print number: 9 8 7 6 5 4 3 2 1

Library of Congress Cataloging-in-Publication Data is available from the publisher.

ISBN 978-1-4625-4765-4 (paperback)
ISBN 978-1-4625-5678-6 (cloth)

We are the intimacy that we seek.

Contents

PART I

PREPARING FOR THE JOURNEY

Introduction

We are the intimacy that we seek.

This book is about cultivating intimacy. It is a guide to walking the path of intimacy in your relationship and in your life. If you feel a lack of connection with your partner and with the world, then you are feeling the call of intimacy. If you seek something deeper and more vibrant in your life, then you are seeking the intimate path. If you yearn to be able to savor what is most precious, to heal what is broken, to hold close what is true and alive, then this book is written for you.

Life can be so unsatisfying in so many ways. We can feel overwhelmed by loneliness, chronically sore from conflict, and fearful of never being truly known and accepted. We can find ourselves at a place in our relationship where we are comfortable, but not close—as if we have traded connection for stability. We miss vibrancy and yearn for deeper connection. This book was written to help set you on the path to rekindling that vibrancy and connection with your partner and with your life.

We are all part of something bigger and more sacred than what we often see as our individual small and lonely selves. We yearn to feel truly known and deeply accepted. We want to be loved thoroughly, just the way we are, including by ourselves. We yearn to stop pretending to be someone or something that we are not; to feel safe in our own skin and treasured in our relationship; to know in our bones that we are not separate from each other, that connection is our birthright, and that we have always been part of something grander and more beautiful than we can imagine.

Whether your relationship is struggling or thriving, there is something in this book for you. There are depths of intimacy and connection that are genuinely fathomless, and we all have an innate wisdom that knows its currents instinctively. This book is intended as a portal to that wisdom. It will help you see relationship as a transformative practice, as it arises out of mindfulness practice, to be enacted and embodied in the ongoing dance between you and your beloved partner. It aims to soften the barriers of your heart and to provide the guidance we need to nurture our intimate connections. I have come to believe that intimacy is the greatest gift that this life has to offer and that intimacy is the only true path to love, wholeness, and unshakable well-being.

The Path to True Intimacy

Our intimacy has always been here, waiting for us to discover it.

> Jamie and Emily have an immediate and powerful connection. They are completely taken by one another and have a beautiful courtship.

When we begin an intimate relationship, the path simply appears. It is broad and wide, smooth and easy. We fall for each other. We fall in love. We are tickled by the perfection of this blessed other who seems to bring us what we have been missing, to be loved for who we really are, to feel safe, cared for, and treasured. In the beginning, the whole thing comes so naturally it is like stepping outside into a beautiful day.

We begin our relationships on the same path as our partner. We walk side by side, openheartedly, lovingly, and passionately. And yet, though beautiful, we find that the intimate path is, ultimately, not an easy one. We discover as we walk it that we have wandered onto the path barefoot and vulnerable. And we learn that the path cuts through untamed wilderness. It is beautiful but wild, comforting yet unpredictable, alive but too vast to be controlled. As our journey deepens, we realize we didn't really read the sign at the trailhead—that if we are to walk this path, we must walk it with bare and tender feet.

Liking all things that are delightfully new, we impulsively and excitedly accept the terms and conditions—not in the mood to trifle with mundane details of future risks—excited to simply begin the journey. So, in stepping on the path, we toss aside our armor and give our heart willingly to this other person. And, for a while, we feel held, seen, and protected by their presence—as if everything will always be okay as long as we have each other.

Jamie and Emily decide to move in together and begin the process of merging their lives.

But, inevitably, on every path of intimacy, there comes a time when the terrain turns a little rougher, the grade gets a little steeper, and the light shines a little dimmer. And through the alchemy of circumstances and inattention we stumble. We get in each other's way, and step on each other's bare toes. We are regularly scratched by brambles, stung by Nature's critters, and tripped by unseen obstacles. And this is how it goes: We walk this path with our person, living long moments when it is light and safe, amidst other moments when it feels darker and more dangerous.

Any authentically intimate relationship will inevitably uncover all of our vulnerabilities—the parts of us that suffer, the places where we have been wounded, our triggers, our insecurities and fragilities—and expose them, naked and undefended. The difference between a relationship of the mundane and a relationship of the sacred is whether we turn toward our woundedness and practice intimacy or turn away and practice separateness. A relationship, whether with another person or a community, will expose our vulnerabilities, and that exposure will either open us up or shut us down, pull us forward into intimacy or cast us into the outer void. There is no in-between space. There is only either intimacy or isolation.

Jamie and Emily are mostly happy. They love each other's company. They are comforted by each other's touch. They share a vision for their future. They laugh at the same jokes and like similar movies. And, as all couples do, they also have disagreements, hurt each other's feelings, and from time to time take each other for granted.

Eventually, perhaps, we start to feel disappointed, hurt, maybe even angry that the headiness of our love hasn't saved us from the subtlety of our suffering—hasn't saved us from our dissatisfaction, our irritability, our wishing it were otherwise, our loneliness, our trauma, our fragility, our vulnerability. So we start to fuss and turn away.

Along the way, we pass other paths that look wider and smoother. Paths that don't include our partner. Paths that don't require our vulnerability. Paths that let us put our protective clothing and sturdy boots back on to keep us safe. We step off the shared path of intimacy and onto an easier path that doesn't ask so much of us. Paths of work and hobbies and TV, Instagram and children, pets and exercise. We begin to diverge. We begin to move, often imperceptibly, in different directions. Sometimes we notice the growing distance early and might step quickly back onto our shared and more intimate path. But, too often, we become lost—we lose each other and the path, and the world gets darker, lonelier, and smaller.

But at least we have our boots back on.

As their relationship continues, Jamie and Emily get caught up in the pressures of life. Emily's job gets more and more demanding, and she has less and less time to devote to their relationship. Jamie finds comfort in friends and hobbies and discovers other ways to fill time without Emily. They both feel so exhausted by their individual paths that when they do find themselves in each other's presence, it more often than not takes the shape of watching TV or scrolling on their phones. As their attention turns away, arguments become more frequent, and cold silences fill the space between their designated seats on the couch.

We begin to miss each other. Though we have settled onto parallel paths that only occasionally intersect, we hunger for intimacy and connection, for knowing and being known, for love and liberation. But how do we find our way back to the shared path that we have lost? And, knowing what we now know, will we be willing to take our shoes off and enter again with bare feet?

Jamie and Emily love each other deeply. They remember the excitement and passion of their early relationship. Nothing terrible has happened, life simply got busy, and yet they find themselves far apart and longing for the closeness they felt at the beginning. Jamie misses Emily but doesn't want to be the first to say it, in case Emily hasn't noticed and doesn't feel the same. Emily misses Jamie but doesn't want their conversation to turn into an argument, so instead of broaching the subject, she finishes her chapter, rolls over, and turns off the light.

The Problem

There is an inescapable problem at the heart of intimate relationships that scares us off, yanks us back, frightens us, and turns us away from the true depth of intimacy that we yearn for and are genuinely capable of. Simply put, the problem is pain. Not just that genuinely walking the path of intimacy is sometimes painful, but that our deepest instinct is to turn away.

Many of us, maybe most of us, get a brief peek at the true gift of real intimacy at the very beginning of a new romantic relationship, when the way is broad and easy. But that's just the entry, where being barefoot is met with soft grasses and smooth earth, exciting conversations, and undiluted attention. When the intimate path inevitably gets more difficult and requires more from our bare feet, we tend to want to find easier paths or to put our boots back on. But the intimate path doesn't respond to tough soles. And we wind up treading on a path that only approximates the intimate path. We are left with something. . . . less.

But, honestly, our experience is that our relationship is still good, still satisfying—sort of. So, we murmur platitudes about how that giddy "falling in love stage" can't last, isn't meant to last, is somehow childish and impractical. I mean, who walks the world in bare feet? Serious grownups wear shoes. We congratulate ourselves on our maturity and realism as we settle into a relationship that is kind of close—but not too close. Secure but not vital. Stable but not rich. Predictable but not transformative. Okay, but. . . . incomplete.

We still know, somewhere deep in our bones, that we are missing something vital to our happiness. Somehow being fully engaged is gone, and we don't know how to get it back. We worry that maybe it wasn't all that real or serious to begin with. So, in its absence, we busy ourselves with the mundanity of life: work, chores, responsibilities, and commitments. We bide our time, distracting ourselves from our looming sense of disconnection and dissatisfaction. We know we are not intimate, but at least we have sturdy shoes.

And thus, because we are shod, because we cannot imagine treading the path with bare feet, there is a gap in our relationship that we cannot seem to close. A distance between us that we cannot seem to bridge. And it is in that gap that we suffer, that we ache, that we yearn and call out, searching for something we can't quite name and can't quite capture. We are strangers to each other. Lonely, misplaced strangers.

> Jamie and Emily have grown apart. They have turned away from one another. They often tell their friends that it feels as if they are "ships passing in the night" rather than romantic partners. They continue to argue and hurt each other's feelings. So, as the easiest solution, they simply interact less. Jamie stops asking Emily when she will be home from work. They stop eating meals together, watch TV in separate rooms, and go to bed at different times.

Maybe we become unkind, withdrawn, angry, dispirited, irritable, sad, and melancholy. We leave one relationship and enter another, hoping to, this time, find what we could not find before, only to discover ourselves once again in the same place—lonely, lost, embattled, wandering through our lives either searching or hopelessly resigned to our dim fate.

The Solution

Fortunately, this gap between us is not our fate. We were born barefoot, and our true nature yearns to be freed. This is where practice comes in. We cannot walk a wild path barefoot with skill and grace unless we are awake, aware, clear, mindful, and lovingly attentive to every step we take. Because every single step we take, every time we place our foot on the earth, it matters.

True love and intimacy are waiting for us below our defenses, below our fearfulness, below our hurt and worries. True love, true intimacy, is not just a destination—it is a journey that we travel arm-in-arm, heart-to-heart, barefoot together. It is a path that we must walk with great and mindful care. It is a path of tenderness and vulnerability, of authenticity and acceptance, of turning toward and meeting all the vicissitudes of this life as partners, friends, and lovers. It is the mindful path of true intimacy.

> Jamie and Emily are acutely aware of the chasm that has developed between them. The distance is palpable, but how it got there is a

confusing mystery. It's scary to reach across the gap, but, at a certain point, it's either that or walk away. And for Jamie and Emily, their relationship means too much to walk away. So, with all their fear and all their courage, they make the first move to turn toward the gap and reach for their partner on the other side.

How to Use This Book

We yearn to be the intimacy that we seek. But we already are the intimacy that we seek. By this I mean that we are born with the capacity for the connection that lives within the pages of this book and the longing in our hearts. Those seeds of love already exist within you. Given that, there are several ways that you can use this book.

This book is divided into three parts that compose the journey of intimacy. In Part I, "Preparing for the Journey," we start at the trailhead and learn the foundational mindfulness practices that equip us with the strategies necessary for walking the path as gracefully as possible. In Part II, "Walking the Intimate Path," we then turn to the ways that we can nurture and strengthen our healthy connection with our partners. Finally, in Part III, "Overcoming Obstacles on the Path," we tackle common roadblocks and look ahead to plan for the challenging and often unexpected twists and turns that our paths can take. So you can read this book cover to cover—start the journey at the trailhead and conclude by savoring the view. In this way, you can build on each section and use the practices to gain momentum for contemplating the next area of your relationship. This option offers you a deep, thorough, and logical exploration of intimacy.

Each chapter contains sections called "Setting the Intention," "Paying Attention," "Skillful Action" and "Mindful Mantra." In "Setting the Intention," we orient ourselves to the intention of the practice we are taking up in that chapter; our intention is the North Star that we use to help us return to the path when we get lost. In "Paying Attention," we actually take up the specific mindfulness practices for the topic of the chapter; these practices will help us to guide our attention to what will be our focus in the endlessly unfolding present moment. In "Skillful Action," having grounded ourselves in present-moment awareness, we consider the words, actions, and attitudes that are most likely to serve the cause of intimacy and connection, given the topic discussed in each chapter. Some of the practices have a journaling component, so set aside a journal to accompany the mindful meditation practice you will soon develop.

You'll discover a "Mindful Mantra" at the end of every chapter. Reciting mantras is a long-established contemplative practice. The point of a mantra is that we can repeat it to ourselves whenever we need it, to orient and inspire us on the path. My hope is that you'll choose to recite one or a few mantras every day as part of a daily ritual. Perhaps you'll turn to them when you can use a little extra guidance. Either way, the practice is to recite the mantra with your whole heart and full attention, letting it wash over and through you, allowing its influence to be both obvious and subtle. We try it on as a practice, and, as always, we each get to decide for ourselves ultimately whether this mantra serves our intimacy practice.

And still, love is not always logical, and we must start where we are. If you find yourself yearning to jump to the heart of where you are feeling stuck, then leap. Each chapter of this book is intended to offer an explanation of the topic and a mindful, skillful way of moving forward. So, if you are seeking particular guidance on managing emotional reactivity, listening more deeply, or addressing health concerns, you can cut right to the chase. Each chapter is its own lesson. In this way, you might find yourself walking a more meandering path, starting from the middle then winding and traversing wherever your heart leads you.

Your Guide on the Intimate Path

In this book it is my hope to guide you along the path of intimacy through *mindfulness*, an authentic practice of paying attention. You will begin with the simple (but maybe not easy) practice of paying deep and loving attention to the ongoing flow of this precious moment. Next, I will introduce a series of gradually deepening exercises that you can do with your partner, starting with the breath and expanding to a more open awareness.

As you continue your practice of couples-based mindfulness, you will expand into the realm of relational mindfulness. This is the ongoing practice of living together, co-creating your shared life: washing the dishes, walking the dogs, raising the children, packing lunches. Then, from the perspective of this ongoing intimacy practice, you will explore much of the sometimes complicated, sometimes difficult, and often wonderful territory of intimate relationships that you have discovered as relationship scientists to strengthen, enliven, and reveal the deep love, joy, and connectedness that is your true home in each other's heart.

So that you might know and hopefully come to trust your guide, let me start by sharing a little about who I am and why a book about the path of intimacy calls to me.

Over the past 25 years, I've come to view relationship as a *spiritual practice*. If you feel wary when you encounter that term in this book, please rest assured that I am not advocating for nor limiting the understanding of a spiritual practice to any one tradition. For me, spiritual practice points most importantly to cultivating a way of being in a relationship as a transformative *practice*. A practice connotes something very different from our culture's usual way of thinking about a good relationship as either something that requires "work" or as something that is, by nature or luck, "good." "Work" is too boring, too mundane, too "pull yourself up by your bootstraps" effortful. And "relationship" as just naturally or luckily good is too passive, too idle, too easily prone to being taken for granted, ignored, and put to the side.

A *practice*, however, is a calling, a lived intention, something that we take up as a way of being. It is a path of transformation, and it connotes a devotion to something larger than ourselves. It is about connection, union, mystery. It is about devotion to an ongoing activity that broadens, softens, humbles, and connects us to our boundlessness. In my experience, there is nothing like a commitment to the path of true intimacy that invites us to turn toward our sometimes dark and painful places to find our way toward wholeness, peace, connection, and grace within the mystery of our humanness.

My sense of the tenderheartedness at the core of intimate connection was cultivated during my doctoral program at the University of Washington by two leaders in the study of couple relationships, Neil Jacobson and John Gottman, and somewhat more indirectly by relationship scientist Andrew Christensen at the University of California—Los Angeles, who encouraged Neil's emphasis on a very Zen-inspired approach to promoting acceptance in couples' relationships that resonated with me. Fortuitously, at around the same time, I was introduced to the psychology of mindfulness and the practice of Zen meditation through a course taught by eminent addiction scientist Alan Marlatt. I have been formally practicing and, for the last 15 years, teaching Zen meditation.

In my role as a professor at Clark University, I've developed and studied the Relationship Checkup, the relationship health equivalent of an annual physical checkup, designed to help prevent relationship distress and to guide treatment of the broken connection at the heart of most intimate couples' suffering. Dozens of published studies and two books have shown that the Checkup is effective in increasing satisfaction, intimacy, and acceptance between partners. I believe the Checkup is so helpful for couples because it deliberately turns partners more mindfully toward one another and their relationship. It shines life-giving attention on the parts of our connection that have started to fade and gather dust, as they did for Emily and Jamie. It offers couples a deeper understanding of one another that is rooted in compassion and works to bridge the distance that has grown between them.

This book is grounded in all that I've learned through my years of work helping couples develop and maintain the intimate connection we all seek. But as much as I've learned from the scientific study of couples, I believe I have learned even more from the hundreds of couples I have worked with over the years in the intensely intimate setting of my couples therapy practice.

It is in this therapeutic context that I have developed my sense of relational intimacy as a genuinely spiritual practice. As Zen teacher James Ishmael Ford is fond of saying, a real spiritual practice plays rough with the ego. And, my goodness, does true intimacy, rooted in openhearted vulnerability, play rough with the ego. It shows us that we aren't always right, that our instincts aren't always helpful, and that we absolutely must be willing to own our missteps and do things differently. When we can let the practice of intimacy soften us and break down the armor that separates, we can discover the depth of connection that is our true home.

This view of relational intimacy as a spiritual practice has grown organically out of the intersection between my decades-long work with couples and simultaneous practice of Zen meditation.

As the Buddhist monk Thich Nhat Hanh says, "We are here to awaken from the illusion of our separateness." Waking up to our interconnectedness is not a luxury; it is our purpose, our path. I believe that the two essential crucibles for waking up are our contemplative practice and our intimate relationships. I have dedicated most of my life to the understanding and practice of both. This book draws on my personal experiences, case examples, current research in the field of relationship science, Zen teachings, and formal meditation practice.

I have also, over the course of my life, fallen in love (more than once), fallen out of love (more than once), and raised wise, compassionate, and beautiful children. I have felt deeply intimately connected, as well as heartbroken and lonely. I have walked this path from one end to the other and back. And the journey continues and deepens. Let me welcome you here, onto this path of intimacy. The Persian poet Rumi once wrote, "Love has inflicted so many pains on me, but that is how my life became blessed." The path of intimacy is not for the faint of heart, but it is worthy and beautiful, and we are blessed by it.

In this book I often use couples, like Jamie and Emily, as illustrations. These couples are an amalgamation of the many couples I have worked with in therapy, and I have changed details to protect the couples' identity and confidentiality. I hope they will resonate with your experiences and help you find your own way on the path to intimacy. I hope more than anything that this book serves you well. I hope you and your person, your love, your partner, come out at the other end of this short, shared journey closer, more intimate, more loving—walking a path together in this lifetime with great and immeasurable joy.

When the ego drops away, love leaps up to catch us.

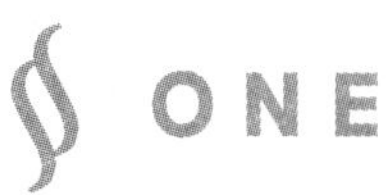

Paying Mindful Attention

THE MOST BASIC FORM OF LOVE

Attention is the most basic form of love.

Please take a moment to deeply consider this trail marker on the path to intimacy. Don't move past it too quickly. Maybe recite it, like a lyric. Think it through thoroughly. Feel into it. Feel where it settles into your body. Feel it in the depth of your bones. Find the truth in it for yourself.

Attention is the most basic form of love. Fully acknowledging that attention is the most basic form of love, we allow ourselves to rest in the intention to enact and embody love. We start with turning our attention to . . . attention.

In my experience, our attention is always on—like a ceaseless beam of light, endlessly flicking from one object to another. The problem is that our attention is untrained, like a new puppy, unruly and with a mind entirely its own. Our attention wanders from thing to thing, topic to topic; we are easily distracted by the shiny or the sharp. Our attention is drawn to our screens and our worries, our tasks and our terrors, our pleasures and our. . . . Look! It's snowing! Haha! I love snow!

Attention is the most basic form of love.

Anyway . . . where were we?

Oh yeah, attention. Right. Attention, by its very nature, wanders.

In Buddhism, this oh-so-human phenomenon is referred to as the *monkey mind*. Our attention and thoughts skitter from branch to branch like a wild and hyperactive monkey. Never settling in any one place for long. Always restless. Always moving.

And isn't it just like this in our relationships? Our attention flickers back and forth and. . . . wanders. Even when our partner is right next to us, or right in front of us, our attention hops about, sniffing here and there. We see and then don't see. We hear, and then don't hear. Even if our partner is talking right to us, even if it is about something dear to their heart, we find ourselves repeatedly distracted—by our own thoughts, our need to respond, our reactivity, our other interests, our responsibilities. . . . our phone.

And, of course, we suffer the reverse. Calling out and yearning to be heard, to be understood, to be seen clearly and known with warmth and care, and yet met with our beloved other's flickering attention, tuning in and tuning out, here and hearing and then gone and daydreaming. It is no wonder that we all carry a certain loneliness, like a lost child who has given up on ever seeing her parents again.

Why is our attention such a fickle thing? Partly it is just the nature of the untrained mind. Monkey mind is our inheritance; we come by it frustratingly naturally. However, I also suspect that our attention is drawn away in the service of our avoidance. Attending to what it is actually like to be this human being in this moment can be disturbingly uncomfortable. Attending to what it is actually like to be relating to this beloved other in this moment can feel intensely vulnerable, scary, and raw.

Because we crave comfort, we turn our attention to whatever our preferred poison is: TV, phone, work, kids, lawn, dishes, drink, or drama. We prefer the familiar confines of our habit-formed stories about ourselves, each other, and the world, lost in the morass of our own thoughts and constructed delusions. Protecting our fragile ego. Writhing in our undigested pain. Preferring the devil we know to the vibrant, unchecked reality of the unfolding moment.

What Is Mindful Attention?

At the heart of this book, at the heart of this practice of intimacy, is the practice of *mindful attention.* Why? Because the practice of mindful attention is absolutely necessary if we are going to deepen our relationships from "close but not too close" to genuinely transformative intimacy. Three of the important qualities that meditation practice confers are (1) increasing the quality of the attention that we bring to our beloved other, (2) stabilizing our hearts so that we can lovingly host our shared vulnerability with courage and grace, and (3) creating the conditions under which we might awaken from the illusion of separateness and experience true intimacy.

Our beloved other needs our loving and undivided attention. Without it, they cannot thrive, they cannot grow, and our relationship with them cannot deepen into genuine intimacy. I am often struck by how vanishingly rare it is for any of us to receive caring, undivided attention. Often, when we are with our partner or even our most precious friend, their attention is lost on their own thoughts and feelings and life circumstances. When we talk to them, they are not really listening to us, but mostly waiting for the opportunity to talk about or go do their own thing. And if we're honest, we're doing the same thing to them. We don't really listen to understand them. We listen to react or for something that reminds us of something we would like to say.

But—and I notice this often with my clients—when someone really gives us their undivided and nonjudgmental attention, we blossom; we are delighted and enlivened and healed by the mindful attention of others. And when intimate partners bring that kind of loving, mindful attention to each other, they come to life in ways that are genuinely beautiful to behold. So this is what I want for you. I want you to learn how to practice bringing your full, open, loving attention to your partner so that you can see for yourself how transformative that can be for your partner, for yourself, and for your intimate relationship.

Mindful Attention as Meditation

Perhaps even more deeply, mindful attention as a *meditation* may be the only effective path to developing our ability to gently host our reactivity with the generosity and spaciousness necessary to genuinely cultivate a safe home for our and our partner's vulnerability.

Almost all people respond with either fight or flight to the cuts and scrapes that are an inevitable consequence of vulnerability on the intimate path. And our fight-or-flight responses are simply deadly to intimacy.

Mindful attention as a meditation may be the only effective path to developing our ability to gently host our reactivity with the generosity and spaciousness necessary to genuinely cultivate a safe home for our and our partner's vulnerability.

Ongoing, dedicated contemplative practice may be one of the only things that systematically and effectively build our capacity to experience our reactive fight-or-flight responses with the clarity and grace that allow us to stay grounded, gentle, and attentive enough to nurture intimacy rather than destroy it when we are upset.

An ongoing, dedicated contemplative practice begins to create the conditions under which we might receive the gift of seeing clearly into our true nature, the gift of awakening from the dream of separateness into the reality of intimacy—intimacy with ourselves, with our partner, and with the whole of the universe. Intimate relationship as a spiritual practice holds the promise of awakening that is at the heart of all contemplative spiritual traditions.

Mindful attention as a meditation comes with challenges. As soon as we sit down and start to pay dedicated attention to our inner landscape, we immediately make contact with how hectic our mind is, how uncomfortable our body is. We notice all the emotions we are experiencing, such as worry, anxiety, sadness, and embarrassment. We notice how difficult it is to keep our attention on the object of meditation (such as our partner's hand or our breath), as our attention repeatedly and unrelentingly wanders from thing to thing.

These challenges are a feature of mindfulness practice and not a bug. It is precisely these challenges that usually turn us away from our true selves and corrode our capacity for intimacy. Yet the stability and kindness of the practice allow us to experience all the complexities of being human. And it is through that experience that we become more lovingly intimate with ourselves and with each other.

The stability and kindness of the practice allows us to experience all the complexities of being human. And it is through that experience that we become more lovingly intimate with ourselves and with each other.

Practicing Mindful Attention with Your Partner

The deep, curious, and loving attention that is necessary for walking the path of intimacy must be cultivated and strengthened so that we can count on it when we most need it in our relationships. So how do we grow our capacity for groundedness, stability, flexibility, presence, openheartedness, and spaciousness? The following mindfulness practices will show you how:

- Hand-holding meditation
- Full awareness of breathing
- Breathing in our partner
- Progressive body scan: Attention to the body
- Sitting with our surroundings: Attention to the senses
- Loving-kindness: Attention to loving our partner and ourself

These mindful attention practices are essential for each barefooted step along the path of intimacy.

HAND-HOLDING MEDITATION

Hand-holding meditation is so simple and yet can be so profound. It has the power to bring you fully into your surroundings and into connection with your partner. It can clear the noxious fog of mundanity or recrimination. Most important, it reminds you that you are not separate from but rather intimately connected to your beloved.

1. To start, find a comfortable seat either facing your partner or sitting beside your partner. The orientation is not so important; you just want to make sure you can comfortably reach your partner's hand, so that neither of you is reaching or overextending your arms.
2. From here, simply hold one or both of your partner's hands, whatever is most comfortable.
3. As you are holding your partner's hands, draw your attention to the full experience of this other being with whom you are sharing this intimate moment. Notice how their hand feels in your hand. Notice the temperature,

the texture, the look. Is the skin slightly sweaty or a little dry? Is the grasp firm or loose? Is the weight heavy or light? Simply notice, without judgment, the sensations.

4. Then, very gently, move your thumb over your partner's skin. What do you notice then? Do you feel a sense of love and affection, missing and nostalgia? Maybe a shiver up your spine or a flutter in your tummy?
5. Take a moment to invite gratitude for your partner's hands. Can you reflect on things that they have done with these hands to demonstrate their love for you? Have they massaged sore muscles, held your hair back when you were sick, brought you food, cradled your babies, walked your pets, taken out the trash, wiped away your tears, written a love letter? Take a moment to reflect on all the acts of service and love that these hands, of this beloved other, have added to your beautiful and complicated life.
6. From here, give your partner's hands a little squeeze. Then smile at each other, hold on or let go, depending on the demands of the next moment. You might also, at this juncture or later in the day, journal about what this experience was like. You can use the questions posed herein to get you started.
7. Rinse and repeat as needed.

A hand-holding meditation is something that can be available to you at almost any time that you are with your partner. You can do some form of the meditation just described or simply engage in a moment of mindful hand-holding or hugging. Whenever you are physically connecting with your partner, bring your full mindful attention to the feel of their touch. Even a brief moment of mindful attention can be of measurable benefit.

FULL AWARENESS OF BREATHING PRACTICE

There are many traditional practices for consciously cultivating your capacity to sustain attention, but perhaps one of the oldest and most thoroughgoing is breath practice. Breath practice is, in its purest sense, the practice of intimacy itself. As you set off on the path of cultivating attention as the most basic form of love, begin by falling in love with the breath.

In traditional Buddhism, the practice of conscious breathing as taught by the Buddha is presented in the Anapanasati Sutta as the discourse on the full awareness of breathing. The practice is simply put:

Breathing in, I know that I am breathing in. Breathing out, I know that I am breathing out.

Though the sutta goes on, in essence this is the true heart of the practice.

What I appreciate about this practice is its simplicity, practicality, and precision. Its simplicity can help you settle directly into it, without overthinking things; just consciously follow the breath. Its practicality is in how readily accessible breath practice is to anyone; the tools of practice—attention, body, and breath—are always carried with you. Its precision is in how immediately breath practice puts you into contact with the ceaseless flow of the moment. In all honesty, everything that there is to be awakened to is already right here in the ongoing flow of the breath. This practice is both elegant and earthy.

1. If you are physically capable of sitting in an upright and dignified manner, then do so. (If you are not physically able to sit upright on a chair or a cushion, you can lie down.) If you are sitting on a chair, place your feet squarely and solidly on the floor and position yourself so that you are sitting very close to the front edge of the chair, so that your weight is somewhat evenly distributed between your sit bones and your feet and so that you are not resting on the back of the chair but sitting up straight.
2. You may notice some arising discomfort in the back, as we are commonly not used to an upright posture, and we are asking our back muscles to do something a little unfamiliar. This discomfort is not a problem and will ease with ongoing practice.
3. Now, place your hands on your thighs, either palms up or palms down, whichever feels most natural. Maybe pull your shoulders up to your ears and then let them relax back and down. You can roll your shoulders up, back, and down two or three times, and then let them relax and settle in alignment with your ears.
4. Let your gaze lower to a comfortable downward angle that you can sustain with ease. Though it is tempting to close your eyes when you lower them, it best serves your practice of being awake and attentive to keep your eyes open and relaxed. All your senses are open, settled, and receptive in this practice.
5. And now, finally, gently gather and shepherd your attention to become intimate with the physical sensation of your breath. The full awareness of breathing is your intention, aspiration, and vow. Take the breath as the beloved, holding it to your bones, weaving it into every fiber of your experience. Breathing in, say silently to yourself, "I am aware that I am

breathing in." Breathing out, say silently to yourself, "I am aware that I am breathing out." Your practice is to attend as closely and lovingly as you can to every micro-moment of the ongoing flow of inbreath and out-breath.

6. Let yourself dissolve into this endlessly arising flow. Breathing in, full awareness of breathing in. Breathing out, full awareness of breathing out.
7. Whatever else arises in your mind or through your fully open senses, simply invite to flow with the ongoing stream of breath. Thoughts arise, and simply allow them to flow gently on the current of the breath, without getting caught by or lost in them. And, when you inevitably do become caught by or lost in your thoughts, simply remember to regard them as particles on the stream of breath and let your attention settle intimately back into the stream, allowing the particles to float freely on their own.
8. When you become aware of sounds, other physical sensations in the body, sensations on the skin, or the things that you can see with your open eyes, invite each of them, as they arise, to join intimately in the flow of the breath. Breathe in and through them, letting them become part of the stream, and return to attentively embodying the flow of breath.
9. If it helps you to remain awake and concentrated, you can count each breath. Count "one" on the inbreath and "two" on the outbreath. Or, say silently to yourself, "in" on the inbreath and "out" on the outbreath. Let the counting or the labeling become one with the flow of breath. Let yourself become the flow of breath entirely, holding nothing back. Your whole life, your whole heart, your whole mind, every single iota of everything that you are, everything that has ever happened to you, everything that will ever happen to you, give it all to the breath. Let the breath carry it. Let it be dissolved in the ceaselessly warm current of breathing in and breathing out.
10. There is nothing here but breathing. There is nothing here but breath. This is attention. This is love.
11. Practice like this for a set period of time. If you are new to meditation and doing it on your own, start with 5 minutes and then build up to 15 or 30 minutes.

The point of setting a specific period of time is to encourage us to stay in our seats, regardless of what is happening, until the bell rings. This intention to stay seated is important because it is virtually guaranteed that we will want to, at some point, escape the container of practice. All the enemies of sustained attention will array themselves against us: boredom, anxiety, unquiet mind, frustration, uncertainty, a sense of failure, yearning to do something/anything else. And these are exactly the teachers whose lessons we must learn, whose intimacy we must cultivate, on our path to truly knowing attention as the most basic form of love. We take our vow to be still and upright for 15 minutes, and then, in the service of that vow, we invite it all—from boredom to yearning for something else—to be intimate with the flow of the breath.

When the bell eventually does ring (whether it felt like mere moments or multiple lifetimes), we take a deep breath, bow to ourselves and all beings, and ready ourselves to stand and move forward into the rest of our lives. Know that progress has been made, even if it is seemingly imperceptible. Your capacity to attend on purpose, fullheartedly, has strengthened. And thus so has your capacity for intimacy and love.

BREATHING IN MY PARTNER PRACTICE

We are often tempted in meditation practice to find a way to withdraw from the world and turn away from others. We are accustomed to armoring ourselves within our sense of separation—imagining that we cannot be known, that we are safely hidden, that everything we are ashamed of can be kept safe and private for now and for always. This is how we have learned to hold our vulnerability.

Fiddling with the solidity of that boundary may simply feel like too much. And this is good and fine and not a problem. The path and practice of intimacy is only meant to be traveled one shuddering step at a time, not to be rushed or pressured or flagellated by "oughts" and "shoulds." As we feel ourselves resisting allowing our partners to enter our skin and bones in this practice of interdependent co-arising breath practice, the practice is simply to notice the arising of that hesitation and to allow it to be breathed in with the same tenderness and love that we are cultivating for every flicker of our endlessly emerging experience. It is enough simply to notice and receive. Nothing requires force. This is an ongoing practice, both utterly complete within each breath and endlessly transforming into wisdom and compassion.

1. Sit facing each other or side by side. Either way, sit in such a way that you can be acutely aware of your partner's presence as part of the experience of the moment.
2. As you settle into your posture and begin to bring your attention to the

physical sensation of breathing, take a few moments to connect intimately with and dissolve into the endless arising of the inbreath and outbreath.

3. Then open your field of awareness to allow the entirety of body, mind, heart, and senses to flow intimately with the breath. In particular, privilege your awareness of your partner's presence. Maybe you can see some part of their body through your partially open eyes. Maybe you can hear their breathing or simply feel their presence more subtly in your field of awareness.
4. However you receive your partner's living presence, breathe them in, opening your heart and pores to include them completely, with no separation, in the intimate arising of the moment. The intention here, as Thich Nhat Hanh says, is to awaken from the illusion of separation. And what does he mean by that? Here, it means to feel into the truth that in this breath, as you fully receive the felt presence of your partner, there is no clear demarcation between this one and that one. Instead, there is simply the whole cloth, utterly inclusive of everything that is you and everything that is your partner, so thoroughly interwoven that it is physically palpable that there is only just this one intimately interwoven fabric—breathing in and breathing out.
5. Sit like this together, breathing each other in for the entirety of the time you have committed to together—until the bell rings or the earth ends.
6. When the bell rings, bow to each other, meet each other's eyes, kiss your partner, lean in, and hold each other for a few breaths.
7. Bow again. Stand up. Move on together into your day.

Moving beyond (but always coming back to) the breath, there are several other mindful practices that can strengthen our ability to direct and sustain our attention. Those include attention to the body, attention to our senses, and attention to love.

PROGRESSIVE BODY SCAN: ATTENTION TO THE BODY

The progressive body scan may be done individually or with a partner. To practice with a partner, you may choose to read the instructions together and then take turns calling out different body parts to attend to, starting at the top and working your way down—that is, from the crown of your head all the way to the soles of your feet.

1. Start in an upright and dignified seated posture. (If you are not physically able to sit upright on a chair or a cushion, you can lie down.) Guide your attention to how your body feels.
2. Notice the points of contact between you and your supports. How do your sit bones feel grounding into your base? What is your experience of the floor? Is it warm or cool? Firm or plush?
3. Next, guide your attention to the very top of your body, the crown of your head. Simply notice. What does the top of your head feel like? What is there to be attended to? Can you feel where your hair is parted? Or, if you are bald like me, can you notice a breeze running over your skin, or the fabric of your hat gently pressing against your scalp? Simply notice, without judgment.
4. Then you move your awareness down, paying exquisite attention to your face—are your eyes tired, dry, squinty, or are they heavy and relaxed? Is your nose stuffy or clear? Is your jaw clenched or slightly ajar? Where is your tongue in your mouth, resting on the bottom or pressing against the top teeth? How do your lips feel against one another? What is there to be noticed in your ears? Can you feel the difference between the tip and the center? Simply notice, without judgment.
5. Continue downward, to your neck and shoulders. You are essentially pouring your attention over your body, like honey, and following the sweet, slow flow, as it drips down your arms, down to your fingertips. . . .
6. Then slowly travel down each vertebra, over your chest, and ribs, and belly. . . .
7. Then follow it still as it slides over your hips, pelvis, and sit bones, and immerses your legs, knees, calves, ankles, and feet, and finally into your toes.
8. At each step of the way, notice all the subtleties, nuances, and sensations that are there to be experienced. Do you notice warmth, coolness, tension, stiffness, pain, ease, openness, relaxation, prickling, flexing, heaviness, lightness, fullness, or expansiveness?
9. As you draw the progressive scan to a close, see if you can feel each of your toes individually.
10. Then guide your awareness to the exact same place you started, noticing how your body feels in your seat. What is the same? What has shifted and changed?
11. Once you have soaked your entire body in your attention, bow and honor the miracle of this physical form that carries us through our entire lives.

SITTING WITH OUR SURROUNDINGS: ATTENTION TO OUR SENSES

There is a relatively new approach to working with children who are overstimulated, overwhelmed, or dysregulated whereby their grownup (teacher, guardian, parent, sibling) helps settle them into the moment by asking them to list three things they can see and three things they can hear. This is a powerful grounding experience no matter how old your inner child has become.

1. To attend to your surroundings, start by finding a seated posture. Maintain a stillness in the body and an upright form throughout the practice, if you can. Bring your awareness to your breath.
2. Then guide your awareness to each of your senses. Notice all that there is to be noticed.
3. Look, notice, and attend to all that you can see. Rather than placing your head on a swivel and looking all around the room, simply hold your head centered and keep your eyes softly gazing down. You might start by focusing on the floor in front of you, the color, texture, and pattern. Notice your own body—your knees and hands and the clothes that you're wearing. As your sight settles, you can expand it to take in the details of your peripheral vision. Can you see a bookshelf or a fan, a painting, or a doorway?
4. Next, attend to the sounds of the world around you. Cars passing on the street outside, the tick of the clock, the hiss of the radiator, the click-clack of dog paws on the hardwood floor as they come to investigate your mindfulness practice. Take several minutes to open yourself to all the sounds of the moment, maybe noticing that your awareness becomes sharper and more discerning with time.
5. Next, attend to touch. You may choose to do an entire body scan, as described in the previous practice, or simply feel what you can feel more holistically: how your clothes feel against your body, how your body feels against its base. You might pay particular attention to places of contact, seat against seat, hand resting on thigh, feet grounded on the floor.
6. Then see if there are any smells in the room. Maybe some subtle notes of your lotion or shampoo, a candle that might be burning in the other room, the freshness of the breeze coming through a window.
7. Finally, attend to taste. This is somewhat more elusive in moments when you aren't eating or drinking something particularly yummy. And yet, take

a few moments to notice what you taste in your mouth. The experience of your tongue, saliva, and teeth can give you an array of stimuli that you often overlook, merely because it is not a typical destination of your attention.

As you practice and deepen this sensory meditation, you will inevitably do less reaching out toward and more simply receiving of the many sensations and perceptions. Let go a bit of your self-referential habit and allow each thing to meet itself. Each sensation is a gift given only to itself. In other words, you begin to realize: *"I" do not hear the tick of the clock; there is only "tick, tick, tick,"* or *"I" do not feel "my" body; there is only sensation arising*. In these brief glimmers where there is only receiving and no receiver, you glimpse the true depths of intimacy.

LOVING-KINDNESS: ATTENTION TO LOVING YOUR PARTNER AND YOURSELF

You can practice loving-kindness meditation by yourself or with your partner, on cushions or while washing dishes, when already feeling loving or when grumpy and agitated. Essentially, you can always practice loving-kindness.

There is an abundance of approaches to loving-kindness, or what is sometimes called *maître* or *metta*, meditations. You can't overdose on loving-kindness; no amount is too much.

1. Start by calling your partner to mind. See if you can visualize them and lovingly hold their image throughout your meditation.
2. Next, simply wish your partner well. You can say, "May my partner be well."
3. Then move on to wishing an array of positive, warm, loving, and healthy experiences for your partner.

   It might sound something like this:

   May my partner feel loved.

   May my partner be safe.

   May my partner be happy.

   May my partner be healthy.

4. Then turn your attention to ways in which you can be loving and supportive toward your partner.

   May I love my partner skillfully.

   May I bring my partner joy.

   May I be a source of healing for my partner.

   May I be a refuge for my partner.

   May I remain curious about my partner.

5. Then, and this is the really tricky, super-advanced, Olympic-level part of the meditation. . . . turn your loving attention to yourself.

   May I be well.

   May I feel loved.

   May I be safe.

   May I be happy.

   May I be healthy.

6. If you haven't abandoned ship yet, continue by cultivating loving intentions for your relationship with yourself.

   May I love myself skillfully.

   May I bring myself joy.

   May I be a source of healing for myself.

   May I be a refuge for myself.

   May I remain curious about myself.

The Heart of the Matter

Intimacy is a practice. At the heart of the intimate path is an ongoing mindful-attention meditation practice rooted in stillness and present-centered awareness. Without some commitment to contemplative practice, the intensity of a genuinely intimate relationship can simply be too much to bear. I encourage you to take up one or two of the mindful-attention meditations as a daily practice, particularly as you make your way through the rest of this book, and for the rest of your life. For all of us who strive to maintain a meditation practice amid busy and sometimes chaotic lives, there will be periods when we are able to be more consistent in our practice and times when it slips away from us. This is part of it. When we notice that we haven't been practicing for a while, we can just sit down and start again. There is something deeply meaningful to starting again, over and over.

To nurture an intimacy beyond separateness, we must dedicate ourselves to a practice of mindfully attending to the relentlessly arising miracle that is this very moment—for ourselves, for our beloved, and for all beings. If the idea of relationship as a mindful spiritual practice calls to you, you can trust that you will find your way. The path always finds those who seek it.

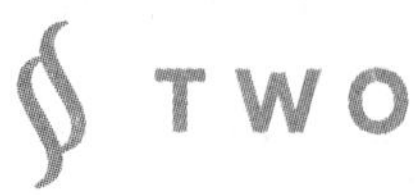

Turning Toward Vulnerability

STRENGTH IN OPENHEARTEDNESS

My experience has been that all intimacy must travel through the gate of vulnerability. And we are vulnerable by our very nature. We are born the physical epitome of vulnerability—entirely dependent on others taking care of our vulnerable selves, protecting our vulnerable bodies, and providing for all of our needs. Throughout our lives, we maintain this physical vulnerability and dependence on others. No matter how physically strong and capable we may be, we are still remarkably fragile: easily injured, susceptible to a panoply of illnesses and disease, subject to the relentless processes of aging, and, of course, thoroughly and irrevocably mortal.

In addition to our fundamental physical vulnerability, our evolutionary heritage has gifted us with an exquisite sensitivity to social rejection. And so we are by our nature incredibly socially vulnerable. Relatively recent research has demonstrated that we experience social rejection literally as physical pain; the same areas of the brain activate in response to both exclusionary and bodily injury. Evolutionary psychologists posit that an exquisite sensitivity to social rejection conferred extraordinary survival benefit, in that being sensitive to even subtle signs of others' displeasure protected individuals from engaging in behavior that could get them banished from the group. And, of course, individuals bereft of a social group are much less likely to survive or procreate. So

All intimacy must travel through the gate of vulnerability.

sensitivity to social rejection kept our ancestors well inside the social fence, where they were safe, had access to resources, and were able to have babies who themselves grew to adulthood and had babies of their own, on down the ancestral lines to us. So we come by our sensitivity to rejection quite honestly.

As a result, we are constantly scanning the social environment for signs that we are acceptable or unacceptable. And, to the degree that we receive signals that we are unacceptable, we experience pain and stress and are *very* highly motivated to return to the good graces of the group. This force of our nature is so strong that we will do things that are clearly against our better judgment, adopt habits that are detrimental to our well-being, and even believe things that are demonstrably false. Avoiding rejection by others is such a powerful motivator that we will do, say, and believe almost anything in its service. The threat of relational disconnection may be at the root of all emotional pain.

So we are, by our most fundamental nature, vulnerable to each other both physically and psychologically.

How We Are Shaped by Others

My theory of intimacy posits that our sensitivity to signs of rejection results in our learning a lot about what is and is not acceptable about us over the course of our lives. In our families of origin, in our interactions with other children at school (mostly middle school, if we're being honest), in basically all social interactions throughout our lives, we have been constantly and relentlessly shaped by the reactions and opinions of others.

Think of all the little and big things that each of us has been teased about, rejected for, judged for, or left out or harmed because of. We carry all of that rejection—as embarrassment, shame, self-criticism, hiddenness, and inauthenticity—as lessons learned.

And what are some of the things we might learn? I'm too short. I'm too tall. I'm too skinny. I'm too fat. I don't have enough money. I'm unattractive. I laugh too loud. It's not okay to be angry, or sad, or even too happy. It's dangerous to love who I love or say out loud that the label I received at birth has always been wrong. I need to be careful how I dress or move. I have to make sure my hair looks a certain way. I can't be too needy. I'm boring. I'm awkward. I'm not funny. I'm not charming. I'm stupid. I'm lazy. I smell bad. I'm too dark. I'm not dark enough. I'm too emotional. I'm not emotional enough. I can't sing. I can't dance. I can't draw. I can't write poetry. I can't write anything. No one wants to hear what I have to say. I'm a failure. I'm worthless.

We learn so many, many lessons about what is acceptable and unacceptable about us. As a result, we do our best, we exert a tremendous amount of energy, to make sure that we only ever show the things about ourselves that are least vulnerable, while relentlessly hiding and protecting the things about ourselves that are most vulnerable.

It is this collection of vulnerabilities, both existential and particular, that we bring to our relationships in the search for love and intimacy, acceptance and care, family and security.

Our innate sensitivity to rejection, our vulnerability to pain, leads us to turn away, to create separation, to believe that we are other. It isn't, however, our vulnerability, in and of itself, that leads to our breakup with the universe. It is our turning away from our vulnerability, our rejection of our vulnerability, our lack of faith in the strength we have to experience the pain and suffering associated with having our vulnerability harmed; it is self-protectiveness (as understandable and maybe even necessary as that is) that turns us away from intimacy. Because intimacy is not for the faint of heart. But all intimacy must travel through the gate of vulnerability.

When Our Vulnerability Is Met

We are also, by our nature, intimate and relational. We are of the nature to seek, form, and nurture relationships. We pair-bond. We form attachments. We fall in love. We love and are loved in turn. Left to our own devices, we will inevitably seek out relationships, including and especially romantic and intimate relationships.

By necessity somewhat oversimplified, my psychological theory of relational intimacy goes something like this. Our usual way of moving around in relation to others requires us to hide and protect as much of our vulnerability as possible. We lead with a false and inauthentic self that has been acquired through hard experience to protect us from the harm of others. But this hiddenness requires active suppression. We have to exert effort to keep our vulnerabilities out of sight and out of reach. But keeping our vulnerabilities hidden is like pushing a beach ball under water. We can do it. We can hide the ball from view. But not without effort. Not without deliberateness and attention and the expenditure of physical and emotional resources. This type of effort is neither pleasant nor infinitely sustainable.

Because inauthenticity is burdensome and effortful, we tend to leak, to slip up, to accidentally let some glimmer of our vulnerability slip through into sight. When this happens, an opportunity for genuine connection emerges. Let's take as an example the quintessential image of a first date. At some point during your evening of striving relentlessly to put only your best foot forward, your date says something genuinely charming and hilarious, and you burst into laughter. Not the polite laughter that you've cultivated to protect yourself, but *that* laugh, the unprotected one, the full-throated, unselfconscious, authentic, real, belly laugh. And now you've done it. You've slipped up. As soon as it happens, you start to feel ashamed and exposed. You try to reel it back in. You brace yourself.

And here, one way or the other, *this moment of vulnerability will be met*, and one of two things can happen: You will either be met well, or you won't.

If the other person reacts in any way that can even vaguely be interpreted as mocking, rejecting, or critical, you will pull it all back in and redouble your efforts to save face and do whatever you can to protect yourself and present only the least vulnerable, most defended self. Getting this reaction decreases the probability of that behavior occurring again in that context. In this case, it is a confirmation of what your history has already taught you—your real laugh is unacceptable and will be rejected by others. And, even more deeply, we reject ourselves—we create separation, pull away from our authentic experience, trying to keep this separate self safe.

But, on the other hand, if the other person responds to your laughter with shared laughter, with delight or warmth, if they brighten and try to keep your laughter alive, then your own delight can be immeasurable. You may also experience relief from both the threat of rejection and the anxiety that exposure created. Any such sequence in which our vulnerable behavior is reinforced by another person results in our becoming freer to engage in that authentic behavior again. In this case, we become more likely and more comfortable releasing our true laughter in the presence of this one special, accepting human being. As the barrier comes down, our true and intimate self is freed. And this is the arising of true relational intimacy, as we begin to feel just a little bit safer being exposed, just a little bit safer being our true and authentic selves.

Events that make us feel safer teach us, at a bone-deep level, that it's okay for us to show up fully. To let down our defenses. To let ourselves be seen for who we actually are. And because suppressing our true authentic self is effortful and separating, as soon as we get any sense that it is okay to let go, we are inclined to want to let go. And doing so genuinely feels like relief. It comes with a kind of "Oh, thank God!" and a desire to lean in. In the analogy, it is that moment of letting go of the beach ball that we have been so effortfully pushing into hiddenness beneath the water. When we release the beach ball, it doesn't just come floating serenely to the surface. It shoots up joyously into the air. Though we may still feel anxious and a little hesitant, having been met well once and having experienced the joy and relief of a moment of acceptance, we start to drop our armor as rapidly as we can. We throw ourselves into intimacy. Into love.

As the barrier comes down, our true and intimate self is freed.

Our true nature wants to shine forth and be known. Intimate events lead to more intimate events. If our partner continues to meet us with warmth and acceptance, we begin to feel safer and safer, and we revel in it. And maybe we return the favor. To the degree that we can share our vulnerabilities and meet each other kindly in that space, we begin the process of weaving a genuinely intimate relationship.

But at a cost.

The Cost of Vulnerabilities

Of course, the price of admission is a kind of psychological nakedness. This comes with its own discomfort. It is not uncommon for people to feel some regret at sharing too much. Some people refer to this as an *intimacy hangover.* Because most of our history has taught us that our vulnerabilities, if exposed, will be harmed, it can feel terribly unsafe to find oneself without armor, or at least with less armor than we're used to having.

So it can require real courage to stay exposed. More often than not, we try to pull back, at least a bit. We hunt around for the bits of armor we left scattered about and try to piece some of it back together, fitting it all back into its familiar places. Some of us resolve this moment of anxiety by literally retreating. We think, "Maybe, if I never see this person again, I can return to feeling safe and unknown." But, in so many ways, it is simply too late. Once exposed, we remain exposed. We cannot slink back into hiddenness. Vulnerability never really becomes invulnerability again.

However, if we want this intimacy, if we are encouraged by this sense of acceptance, we will find ourselves pulled further toward relationship, creating ways to spend more and more time inside this bubble of acceptance and intimacy.

Because vulnerability never returns to invulnerability, now we must learn how to navigate this delicate path of intimacy with another vulnerable, fallible human being.

Both are made vulnerable, and both are navigating intimately close emotional and physical proximity. Figuratively and, at times, literally naked with one another, we cannot help hurting each other. Mostly by accident. Mostly thoughtlessly, without malice, out of ignorance, lack of skillfulness, blindness, reflexivity, reactivity.

The real price of admission is that we enter into a relationship in which this carefully cultivated intimate other becomes the one person in the world who can hurt us the most deeply. Our intimate partner becomes the person who, through no fault of their own, stings our vulnerability the most frequently. They inflict pain, hurt, injury and disappointment, misunderstanding and confusion.

To our partner, in turn, we become the person who most frequently steps on their toes, disappoints them, pushes their buttons, stings them—in terms of raw frequency, more than most and, probably, sometimes more than anyone. Although we commit to moving with care and gentleness, things will get bumped and broken.

The cost is that, after falling into intimacy, we must maintain it right there in the heart of our buttons, our frailties, our insecurities, our low self-esteem, self-criticism, and reactivity.

Falling into love is effortless and delightful. Falling into intimacy is simple, if counterintuitive. But then walking the intimate path? Well, that's where the rubber really hits the road. That is where the real practice of intimacy begins.

Setting the Intention to Turn toward Vulnerability

In Zen and in our intimacy practice, we are regularly reminded of the existential truth that we are, by our very nature, vulnerable. Each of us is vulnerable to the inescapable effects of aging; the inevitability of illness, death, and loss; and our embeddedness within the law of cause and effect. There is no escaping any of this. We are of the nature to be vulnerable.

We acknowledge this shared vulnerability together so that we can support each other in not turning away from our common humanity. So that we might, together, turn toward each other and allow our nature to be our nature, with compassion and grace. Ultimately, it is by turning toward that we invite true intimacy.

Inviting True Intimacy

An *intimate* relationship is a very particular kind of relationship. It requires clear-sightedness and intention. As you learned in Chapter 1, we must deliberately set ourselves on the path of intimate relationship as a practice. It does not unfold naturally any more than the path of awakening unfolds naturally in the absence of intentional and committed practice. So, for most couples, though they may begin with the easily-fallen-into type of intimacy, with time they begin to turn away from each other in an effort to limit their exposure to the intensity of true openhearted vulnerability. They eventually settle into a kind of emotional détente in which they find an emotional distance at which they can be maximally comfortable and minimally exposed: close, but no closer.

Of course, that doesn't really work. When we seek comfort by protecting ourselves from our partner, we still experience our vulnerability, we still hurt, we still experience the pain of being stung. We just keep it to ourselves, encase it in a toxic shell of self-pity, and lose ourselves in the space between the Scylla

The spirit of relational practice is noticing the desperate urge to protect our hearts, to turn away or attack, and choosing instead the discomfort of stillness and of turning toward with care and courage.

and Charybdis of withdrawal and attack, fight and flight, the cold shoulder and the hot insult.

But it is by *turning toward* that we invite true intimacy.

In an ordinary relationship, we continue to turn away. But in a truly intimate relationship, in a relationship intentionally set on the path of intimacy, we do not turn away. Like recalling together our shared existential vulnerability to aging, illness, death, and causality, the practice of relationship helps to call us to meet with compassion the facets of ourselves and the truths of the human experience from which we have come to instinctively withdraw. We stay. We lean in. We turn toward. We open our hearts, more and more. We encourage ourselves to know ourselves deeply and clearly, in all our flawed glory. We orient toward knowing our intimate partner deeply and clearly, in all their flawed glory.

So the spirit of relational practice is choosing the path of fearlessness and courage, the path of staying with the raw humanness that we would otherwise turn away from. Yet at the same time it is a path of gentleness and care and commitment to tenderness. Therefore, it is a practice of noticing the desperate urge to protect our hearts, to turn away or attack, and choosing instead the discomfort of stillness and of turning toward with care and courage.

We make a promise to ourselves and to each other, a vow to discover and notice where and how we separate from vulnerability, and we nurture our intention to turn toward and become intimate with vulnerability.

Paying Attention to Vulnerability

So how do we actually engage this practice in our relationship on a day-to-day, moment-to-moment basis?

As I noted before, this is a practice of presence (which, in this case, necessarily emphasizes not turning away) and attention. When we say that attention is the most basic form of love, we perhaps usually picture ourselves paying more attention to our partner from a place of calm and loving benevolence. If we're honest with ourselves, we might notice that we imagine providing this kind of loving attention from a place of power, with us in the *up-power role* and our partner in the "needing attention," *down-power role*. Attending lovingly and actively to our partner is at the heart of how we nurture a sense of loving and being loved.

However, this is not exclusively what I am pointing to in this spot. I am also pointing to the much more emotionally challenging practice of paying close attention when we are *not* calm but are instead very upset and frighteningly down-power. It is under these much more intense circumstances that "attention is the most basic form of love" becomes a true practice of intimacy. And, of course, this begins with the practice of *not* turning away, precisely when every fiber in our being is pulling us to do so.

NOT TURNING AWAY

This practice of attention involves turning toward and paying close attention to what your vulnerability feels like in your body and in your heart, and what arises in your mind. At this point, you are practicing attention and stillness, and this attention and stillness is enough.

The practice is straightforward. Simply reflect quietly or write your answers in your journal:

- Where do I experience my vulnerability in my body?
- What does it feel like exactly?
- Can I feel the constriction that might be myself protecting itself without judgment or shame?
- What are the thoughts that are arising in my mind?
- Are they familiar?
- What happens when I believe them?
- What happens when I allow myself to be less certain?
- When feeling the discomfort of vulnerability, what do I want to do? Leave? Change the subject? Lash out?

All of this inquiry is for the sake of noticing, exploring, and getting to know your own and your partner's experience of vulnerability without judgment, with acceptance and compassion. Sometimes turning toward is simply not turning away.

Skillful Action: Practicing Vulnerability

Once we have set our intention and then deeply engaged the practice of attention, we can experiment with engaging in skillful action. How do we put turning toward intimacy with vulnerability into practice?

As we get to know the contours of our vulnerability with determination and patience, we begin to free ourselves from our habitual action patterns and open the possibility of moving differently, maybe even more skillfully, right in the midst of feeling vulnerable.

As we get to know the contours of our vulnerability, we begin to free ourselves from our habitual action patterns and open the possibility of moving more skillfully, right in the midst of feeling vulnerable.

THE VULNERABILITY TRIO: BE, SAY, ASK

As you begin to notice that your instinct is to shut down or run away, instead try the following.

1. Practice simply staying present and allowing yourself to receive the experience of vulnerability. Committing to one or more of the mindful attention practices in Chapter 1 and making them a regular, daily practice is essential to your growing ability to experience your own reactivity with stability and clarity. An ongoing practice is also the necessary foundation upon which everything else in this book is built. The practice here is to simply be with uncomfortable urges, to sit in nonjudgment and notice what comes up. This practice of stillness is enough.
2. You can also experiment with communicating about your experience of vulnerability. Maybe say to your partner something like, "I'm feeling pretty exposed and vulnerable right now, and I'm trying to stay present."
3. You might invite your partner to share their experience of vulnerability with you. You might say something like, "My love, can you share with me what is feeling vulnerable right now?" And then you can meet whatever your partner shares with loving attention and understanding.

Of course, all of this is much easier said than done. And you will, at first especially, not feel confident or skillful. But if your intention is transformative practice, then you must set out on the path, even shakily and unsurely. We dive much more deeply into how we might engage skillful practice in each of the remaining chapters in this book.

The Heart of the Matter

Vulnerability is not for the faint of heart. It is not something we achieve once and can then rest. It is a practice. And, like any true practice, it will play roughly with the ego. But, also, like any true practice, it will, if we let it, reveal to us to our true selves, our strength, our interconnectedness, our worth, our home, our boundlessness. If we want true intimacy, we must practice turning toward our vulnerability and our partner's vulnerability with attention, acceptance, and an unwavering commitment to kindness and care—for ourselves, for each other, and for all beings.

Mindful Mantra

When I am stung, may I be stung with grace.
When I am hurt and angry, may I not seek comfort in separation.
May I hold this pain and breathe into this anguish.
May I keep my heart open, be still, and do no harm—to myself or my beloved.
May I turn toward my own ache of vulnerability with mercy.
May I turn my loving attention to my dear one. So that I might hear their cries, touch their hurt, honor their pain—bear witness and offer up compassion for us both.
May I walk the path of intimacy with openness and courage.

PART II

WALKING THE INTIMATE PATH

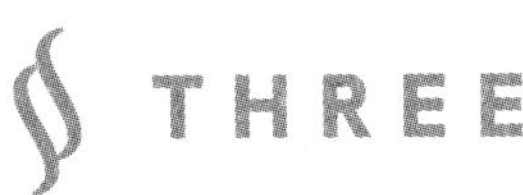

THREE

Being and Seeking a Safe Harbor

THE ATTACHMENT TEETER-TOTTER

Though intimate relationships are woven from many threads, one of the most important and fundamental involves *attachment*. The adult attachment system is a concept from psychology that helps explain how our early childhood experiences shape the way we form and maintain close emotional bonds and relationships as adults. In essence, how our parents cared for us has an impact on how we care for others. This is particularly evident in our most intimate relationships, in which power dynamics can exacerbate patterns of how we relate to one another. This chapter delves into the adult attachment system as it is conceptualized in psychology, how it functions in long-term intimate relationships, and the role that understanding the attachment system plays in navigating the path of true intimacy.

As with all things on the path of intimacy, attachment is about turning toward and receiving—turning toward each other when we are at our most vulnerable and receiving that vulnerability as a secure and safe harbor. This chapter is about the relational practice of taking and providing refuge during life's many storms.

The Evolution of Attachment

In human beings, the attachment system initially evolved between parents and their children. It's fairly easy for us to understand the survival value that accrues to our species (and other mammals) from the extraordinarily tight and sacrificial bond that forms between parents and children. Parents whose attention is strongly oriented toward the care and well-being of their offspring have offspring who are much more likely to survive to become parents themselves.

Any of us who have experienced the strength of that parent–child bond know how viscerally deep and instinctual it is. It is magnetic, effortless, irresistible, and, most apropos of the fundamental basis of practice, it is constructed entirely from the strength of our attention.

As the attachment system evolved, attachment bonds emerged between mating pairs. Obviously, this conferred significant survival value on the species because mates who are powerfully connected emotionally tend to have offspring who are more likely to survive and have their own children. Intense attachment bonds are perhaps the most valuable part of our inheritance. There are few more powerful forces in the human experience than the emotional connection between an attachment pair.

So, in short, the first form of attachment to arrive over the course of our evolution was this irresistible love we have for our children, followed by this same kind of irresistible love for each other.

The Development of Attachment Styles

Attachment styles develop from the ways our caregivers respond to us when we are in distress. Though our emotional connection to our caregivers is in some ways always there, it is most powerfully activated when we are suffering. For example, when, as infants, we cried, the ways our parents responded communicated something fundamental about those parents' availability and responsiveness to our suffering, and therefore taught us a bone-deep lesson about our safety and worth. However, not all parents are equally responsive.

The image that I often use is of a child who wanders around the corner to play and, while happily playing, falls down and scrapes a knee. This moment of hurt is the crucial moment, because, in pain, the child instinctively turns to seek out the care and solace of their caregiver. If the parent is present and responds with attention, care, and warmth, then the child learns that the world of important others is responsive and reliable. If that attentive response is common and, importantly, more common than not, then the child learns that others are not just comforting, but predictably so, and develops what we call a *secure attachment style.*

However, if the parent is either gone, distracted, or in some other way inattentive, then the child learns a different lesson altogether. Sometimes what the child learns is that the world of important others is unreliable, especially if their parent's presence is unpredictable, meaning sometimes present and attending and sometimes not. In those cases, the child develops what is called a *preoccupied* or *anxious–ambivalent attachment style*, in which they become much less willing to comfortably explore their world and much more inclined to stay anxiously close to their parent an effort to make sure they don't lose that parent's attention again in a time of need. So, in this case, you get a child who essentially clings to the parent, is difficult to soothe, and is much less comfortable exploring a world that can at times be painful.

In other cases, when the child seeks comfort, the parent is consistently unavailable and unresponsive. In those cases, the natural human need to seek the comfort of others when suffering is simply extinguished, and the child develops what we call a *dismissive–avoidant attachment style*. Basically, the lesson they learn is that others simply do not care and cannot be relied upon and, therefore, their suffering is theirs alone to bear. When in need, it no longer even occurs to them that others might be a source of aid or comfort.

Finally, in the most distressing cases, when the child seeks comfort, the parent responds harshly and painfully. Maybe the child hears something like "I'll give you something to cry about" or "Suck it up and walk it off" or "Don't be a baby; big boys don't cry." In those instances, the child learns that it is actually shameful or frightening to bring their pain to others and develops what we call a *fearful–avoidant attachment style*. It is important to note that in this attachment style, the natural human urge to seek the comfort of others when suffering is not extinguished but simply suppressed. And there is, therefore, still a palpably deep yearning for connection underneath a strong, earned fear of rejection. They may believe, "I want to be held, but I am ashamed."

An important thing to note here is that all of the attachment styles derive from a moment in which there is a power differential between the one who is seeking comfort and the one who is providing comfort. It is necessarily the case that the one who is seeking comfort and security is approaching the other from a place of need, and needing or wanting someone's care is, by its nature, a down-power position in the relationship. Therefore, in meeting that, the person who provides comfort and reassurance enters that moment of relationship from a somewhat up-power position.

And herein lies the complexity of attachment relationships between romantic partners. The inherent power differential within *comfort seeking* and *comfort providing* is not so much an issue when the relationship is parent–child, because in many ways the parent–child relationship is defined by the parent being in the up-power position and the child necessarily being in the down-power position. However, between equals in an ongoing long-term intimate relationship, power differentials create complexities that can at times be incredibly difficult to navigate.

Power Differentials in Attachment

One of the things that I often say to couples is that "intimacy doesn't flow uphill." By this I mean that when my partner meets my vulnerability well, I feel safer with her, but she doesn't necessarily feel safer with me—because she didn't make herself vulnerable to me. As noted in the previous chapter, if the partner who expressed vulnerability feels well met, that person is more likely to feel safe being their authentic vulnerable self with that partner and more likely to express their vulnerability and desire for comforting again in the future.

The partner who is providing comforting, however, is not also simultaneously seeking comfort. So they do not experience the same degree of vulnerability nor receive the same opportunity to experience feeling comforted, and therefore they don't experience the same potential increase in intimate safety. Thus the strongest experience of building intimate connection happens in the direction from power-down to power-up, and not as thoroughly in the direction of power-up to power-down. Thus intimacy doesn't flow uphill.

I should note here that it does feel good being the person who provides comfort and who is sought out for comforting, and the comforter does experience an overall increase in intimate connection at the relationship level. However, at the individual level, that person has not taken the same risks in terms of exposing their vulnerabilities as the other.

In a truly intimate relationship, intimacy must be bidirectional. It cannot get stuck in a power differential. Ideally, each partner must feel free and invited to seek the security and comforting of the other when they are feeling unsettled, triggered, frightened, heartbroken, or just spent and wounded by the vagaries and vicissitudes of life. That means that the power differential inherent to attachment relationships has to remain flexible and dynamic, moving up and down in both directions, like a teeter-totter.

When our partner is hurt and needing comforting, we are called to step up into an attachment figure position so that we can provide that secure base. But when we need comforting and soothing, we have to step down into a position of greater vulnerability inherent in authentic comfort seeking. And our partner, in turn, must step up to provide that comforting secure base in an effective way. In an ideally functioning intimate relationship, there is an easy flow as each partner steps into and out of the secure-base position with ease and skill. Keeping the axis greased is of utmost importance.

Intimacy doesn't flow uphill.

The Flow of Attachment Seeking and Attachment Providing

Perhaps one of the bigger threats to a truly and dynamically intimate relationship is the potential for the attachment power differential to become unbalanced or even get stuck, such that one partner is perpetually in the up-power position and the other in the down-power position. This can happen for several reasons.

For example, some of us have learned over the course of our lives that being vulnerable and expressing vulnerability are particularly fraught and dangerous, that expressing vulnerability risks censure, mocking, and rejection. We can learn to fear vulnerability so thoroughly that we actually hope to never have to reveal or express that vulnerability to anyone else. When that is the case, we sometimes also find other people's expression of vulnerability incredibly aversive, and so we are unable to receive that vulnerability in warm and comforting ways. With no ability to experience and offer our vulnerability to others, and no capacity to remain openhearted and available to receive the gift of others' vulnerability, intimacy is simply unavailable to us in our relationships and in our lives.

However, at other times, our yearning for intimacy in combination with the fear of expressing vulnerability manifests as a willingness and even desire to receive the vulnerability of others and to be sources of warmth and caring to others; yet at the same time we remain uncomfortable and unwilling to actually express any vulnerability of our own in that relationship.

When this is the case, we create relationships that are defined by a kind of *unidirectional false intimacy*, in which one person is almost always the comforter and the other the comforted. Relationships that are stuck in this inflexible pattern are almost always dissatisfying and result in accumulating resentment on both sides. The person in the perpetual down-power position comes to resent always being the only vulnerable one and never getting to be the one who is strong and capable of taking care and providing comfort. The down-power member of the couple also may come to feel "always broken," "too needy," or even basically incompetent. The person in the perpetual up-power position, in turn, feels more and more lonely and unknown and resentful of having to be the one who always listens and is never heard, provides comfort and is never comforted.

This unbalanced relationship pattern is unfortunately likely to emerge in a relationship in which one partner becomes chronically ill, either physically or mentally. These relationships can easily slip into a caregiver–care receiver relationship pattern. The partner who is experiencing that illness is, in those moments, by definition, also experiencing greater ongoing vulnerability in the relationship and is in greater need of care and comforting. The power differential inherent in caregiver–care receiver moments is in some ways unavoidable; however, the fact that one partner is perhaps momentarily needing more frequent care does not necessarily mean that that partner cannot also provide care, support, comfort, and attachment security to the other. We explore this issue in much more depth in Chapter 15.

Sometimes, though, the partner who is not currently ill can feel as though they can't lean on their unwell partner and therefore may become reluctant to seek comfort and soothing out of an overabundance of seeming compassion and unnecessary guilt. It is particularly important for couples who are experiencing a period of illness to be encouraged to maintain the flow and flexibility of their attachment connection such that both partners are able to receive the gift of the other partner's vulnerability and the need for care. The partner who is ill wants and needs to feel needed, strong, and still called upon to provide nurturing and soothing. And the partner who is momentarily well wants and needs to know that they can seek their partner's strength and support without feeling like they are overburdening the other. Consider this mantra: *On my deathbed, as I gratefully receive your loving care, I can still hold your hand and comfort your heart before the lights turn out and we drift off to sleep.*

Interrupted Flow

Let's look at Beth and Tom, who epitomize a pattern in which the attachment system does not flow, even though they love each other very much.

> Tom and Beth had met many years earlier, fallen in love, and gotten married. Some years into their marriage, Tom developed some significant health issues, resulting in the loss of his left leg below the knee and sometimes significant pain and periods of being quite unwell. When Tom first became ill, Beth naturally and compassionately stepped into a caretaking role. Tom needed the care and deeply appreciated the extra help, as well as her kindness and sympathy.
>
> As sometimes happens when one partner develops a more chronic condition, however, Beth found herself stuck in an up-power position as the caretaker and started to feel that she shouldn't really add to Tom's burdens with her own troubles—small or big. Tom, on the other hand, became stuck in a down-power position, receiving care but no longer really finding himself called on or motivated to exert the energy and effort to provide care. Though he could go to Beth when he was upset and be comforted by her, somehow it just didn't feel the same anymore—less satisfying, like something was missing, and he could feel the closeness between them fading. Beth, though she loved Tom and appreciated being able to care for him, began to feel increasingly lonely and separate, that something in their partnership had been lost along the way.
>
> The caretaker–care receiver pattern had settled so naturally into their relationship that it was imperceptible to them. Though they lived it out every day, they could not see it and therefore had no perspective from which to choose to do things differently. In therapy, they were able to start to see this pattern of stuckness from a new perspective, with compassion for the unfolding of circumstances that brought them to it.

As they came to know it more clearly, Beth was able to see that she was holding back in seeking comfort from Tom and to recognize that Tom was still not only capable but eager to provide that comfort to her. For his part, Tom was able to see how he had fallen out of the habit of doing his own active and loving caretaking of Beth, both asked for and unasked for, and found that he genuinely appreciated stepping back into the role of soother, confidant, and comforter for her. As their attachment teeter-totter started to flow back and forth more smoothly again, they found they were once again experiencing the deep and sweet connection that had always really been at the heart of their union.

As Beth and Tom illustrate, we must wake up and attend to the flow of attachment seeking and attachment providing that is integral to a healthy and well-functioning intimate relationship between loving adult partners. And we must realize that part of waking up is becoming more and more attentive to and sensitive to the flow of ongoing vulnerability and support within ourselves, within our partners, and within our ongoing relationship.

We must wake up and attend to the flow of attachment seeking and attachment providing that is integral to a healthy and well-functioning intimate relationship.

Setting the Intention to Seek and Provide Comfort

When our beloved other comes to us sad, scared, and brokenhearted, even though we ourselves in that moment, in our empathic and compassionate resonance, are also sad, scared, and brokenhearted, we must open our hearts even wider, feel that depth of heartache even more vividly, acutely, consciously, and wakefully. We must step up to receive our partner warmly and compassionately into our arms with love and acceptance in that place in which we are all suffering beings calling out and receiving the loving embrace of each other.

Equally, when we are brokenhearted, discouraged, confused, lost, and just plain beaten down by life, we are called to wholeheartedly embrace the practice of receiving intimately our own brokenheartedness and offer up our hearts to the universe and to our beloved other. To make a gift of our hearts as they truly and authentically are, to not be hidden or withdrawn or stingy with our own fragility, need, yearning, and loss. For this is the place of true intimate connection between partners as we meet each other and hold each other's openhearted vulnerability and see each other as simultaneously both fragile and boundless.

Paying Attention to When We Need to be a Safe Harbor (Up-Power Position)

So how do we make a practice out of being a good and flexible attachment figure to our partners? As with all things, this begins with cultivating our attention so that we are maintaining a connection to and a sense of our partner's emotional tone in any given moment. An important thing to know is that the attachment system is not always activated and that it really only activates when we are feeling particularly stung or rattled. That means, for the most part, on a moment-to-moment, day-to-day basis, that we are simply being each other's partner, connected heart-to-heart, but not necessarily being called on to actively provide the security and comfort of an attachment figure. Thus part of attentiveness is attentiveness for moments of upset to the normal rhythms of life.

So the first part of the practice, as always, is simply paying attention. Refer to the practices in Chapter 1 for ways to practice mindful attention. Make them part of a daily routine.

Skillful Action: Being a Safe Harbor

The second part of the practice arises when we do notice that our partner is acutely suffering, because this is the moment we are called on to step into our role as their source of security, and this is often more emotionally challenging than we might assume. For example, sometimes, if we're lucky, our partner will come directly to us when sad, hurt, lonely, or afraid and actively seek out the comfort of our arms. However, at other times, our partner might express their suffering by getting quiet or withdrawing, or they might cover it up with busyness or humor. In those moments, it is our practice of loving attention that helps us notice that our partner is having a hard time coming to us with their pain. Attention to our interwovenness helps us notice that when our partner is upset, suffering, or in pain, we can feel it directly in our own bodies and minds.

The practice of skillful action as our partner's attachment figure is to notice when the vulnerability of their pain is making them hesitant to seek comfort, so that we can go to them and actively provide the comforting presence that they may need. Partners with less secure attachment styles, particularly more avoidant attachment styles, may choose to protect their vulnerability by withdrawing or hiding their pain.

Skillful action is whatever we can do to show them that they are safe with us, that it is okay to come to us with their pain, and that we will try to always meet them with love, compassion, and support. If they will not come to us, then we will go to them. We will notice that they are upset and hurting, and we will show them that we care, express our love and support, and do what we can to alleviate their pain. And, even if we cannot make it all better, we will keep them company and let them know with our loving presence that we are their safe place and their harbor in the storm.

For some others, the vulnerability of suffering hides behind a protective shield of anger. One of the more difficult moments to show up skillfully as our partner's romantic attachment figure is when our partner's suffering emerges as some form of anger, whether in a low-intensity form, such as simple fussiness, or a more high-intensity form, such as frustration, open anger, and even rage. Our instinctual, habitual response is to meet fussiness with fussiness, frustration with frustration, anger with anger, and rage with rage, or to respond to all forms of anger expressions with fear and withdrawal.

In this case, the practice challenge is to remain still and upright in our receiving of our partner's angry energy, such that we are able to see clearly through the anger to the heart of the suffering it is rooted in and thus to hold our compassionate heart open and to move in relation to the deeper pain rather than simply reacting to the veneer of anger. Anger is addressed in detail in Chapter 9.

Our partner's anger is always going to sting, and some form of reactivity is always going to arise. The point is not to attain some superhuman state of unassailable equanimity but to meet our own reactivity with stillness, familiarity, and openheartedness so that we might remain other-oriented. This is where we really rely on the strength of our ongoing meditation practice, because this requires the practice of being intimate with the flood of emotions and bodily sensations that will be arising for us in the moment.

If we are not deeply familiar with our own intense emotional experience, and if we have not cultivated a capacity to host that experience with all of its heat and intensity, then we will be completely at the mercy of our own reactivity and will be unable to deliberately and gracefully step up to meet the moment as a safe harbor and place of refuge. So we rely on what we have been cultivating in the practices described in Chapter 1.

Again, here, the practice is to notice what arises for us as we first encounter the heat of our partner's anger. Then, in that noticing, to lean in consciously and deliberately and open up to receiving the full intensity of that experience without turning away—to breathe into it. As we practice hosting the fullness of our experience, we are then able to engage in the practice of looking deeply to feel for the pain and suffering at the root of our partner's anger and to bring forth our compassionate heart and allow ourselves to become a safe harbor. This is why, again, a regular meditation practice is vital to the work we are doing in this book. It endows us with the grace to engage in skillful action in the midst of our own strong emotions.

For some of us, the emotional challenge will be that meeting anger makes us want to fight back; but for others, and this is not at all uncommon, the emotional challenge is that our partner's anger makes us feel as if we are in trouble. In this case, we instinctively slip into a down-power position, in which all of our behavior is in the service of either trying to get out of trouble or trying to escape. The issue here is that if we slip into this down-power position, even our attempts to make our partner feel better will fall short, because we are essentially still leaving them alone with their own suffering, and, having taken their anger too personally, we've made the moment about us and our comfort, rather than about tending to our partner's pain.

To tend to our partner's pain, the practice challenge is to develop our capacity to host our own discomfort, such that we can remain oriented toward the well-being of others. This will be a natural outcome of an ongoing mindfulness meditation practice.

Tending to our partner's pain does not mean that we ignore the form that our partner's anger takes in that moment. Though the first step forward should always be curiosity about, and validation of, the pain that our partner's anger is rooted in, the second step can begin with naming any hurtful form that the anger might have taken. This need not come from a scolding place but more from a place of vulnerability and calling forward our partner's inherent compassion toward us. You might say, "Sweetheart, I know that you are in pain, but it is hard for me to be here for you when you are lashing out in hurtful ways. Can we take a few minutes to breathe and then talk about this again?"

THE STEPS TO BEING A SAFE HARBOR

How might you step into the up-power position and meet your beloved's needs?

1. First, notice when your partner is suffering and breathe them into your heart. Using the growing sensitivity that you are cultivating in your meditation practice, begin to cultivate an awareness of the ways that your partner shows that they are hurting. Do they get quiet when they are upset? Do they complain? Do they become irritable and short? Do they withdraw? Whatever it is, learn to notice it with the compassion that arises from knowing that their pain and yours are not separate and that you have felt and will feel again just the way they are feeling now.
2. Notice how you feel in your body when your partner is upset. Where do you feel any tension or upset in yourself? Notice the thoughts that come up. Is there any judgment or defensiveness arising? Emotionally, do you also feel upset when your partner is upset? Do you worry that you're in trouble, or does your partner's upset feel kind of scary? Just notice what is arising for you without judgment and allow your experience to just be without struggling to change it. Know that the upset you are feeling is your own resonance with your partner's pain.
3. Remember the harbor's vow. Remind yourself of your commitment to be there for your partner when they are hurting. Feel yourself turn your inner compass toward your partner and open your heart's arms to hold and soothe them. Nurture an attitude of caretaking, soothing, and encouragement.
4. Let your partner know that you see that they are suffering and that you care. You might say, "Oh, sweetie, you're really upset. That totally makes sense to me. I'm here to help in whatever way I can. Do you want to talk about it? Do you want me to just keep you company? Is there something I can do that would be helpful?" Hold them in your arms.

5. Remember that the experience that you want to create for your partner is one in which they feel safe with you when they are upset, they feel cared about, and they feel encouraged.
6. Breathe in your partner's upset and breathe out your gift of comforting while you do whatever is called for in your role as safe harbor. Listen, reflect, validate, encourage. No matter the hurt or disaster, let your partner know they are loved.

Paying Attention to When We Need to Have a Safe Harbor (Down-Power Position)

The other side of the teeter-totter is that we clearly and deliberately also need to cultivate the courage to step down into the vulnerability of seeking comfort. This will be easier for some of us than for others. Those of us who were raised with a secure base and have developed a secure attachment style may be most likely to feel reasonably safe approaching our partners from a place of vulnerability and need.

However, for those of us who have been rejected or punished for being vulnerable in our attachment relationships, the need for comforting will be experienced as a kind of fear or shame, and though we yearn for the warm embrace, it may be virtually impossible for us to approach directly and ask clearly.

Some of us will freeze, some of us will withdraw, and some of us will develop indirect and potentially confusing ways of trying to signal our need for comforting without revealing our fragile selves. This fearful–avoidant attachment style is unfortunately common for men (though not exclusive to men) who have been raised in a culture of toxic masculinity in which we are regularly and actively punished for any signs of weakness or vulnerability. It is not surprising, then, that many men have extraordinary difficulty directly and clearly expressing their need for soothing and comfort to their intimate partners.

This is an essential point of practice and not something to be judged, condemned, or vanquished in any way. When we discover that it is fear that arises in relation to our beloved other when we are feeling pierced and broken by the harshness of life, our practice, as always, is to turn toward, open up to, and embrace that fear—to first create a safe harbor for our own tender hearts and then to take that fear and trembling and offer it up, as the gift that it is, to the one who has promised to be our refuge and secure base.

Others of us may discover that our style is more classically avoidant and dismissive and that what arises for us when we are hurting is a sense that others will not care and cannot help. We come by this cynicism quite honestly, and the causes and conditions of our lives taught us this lesson before the age of choice. And yet, the practice of true intimacy requires that we allow the world to teach us a different lesson. Again, first in our practice we must begin the process of creating our own safe harbor for our pain and, especially, for our need to be held. And then, as difficult as it will be, we must risk allowing someone else to see us and meet us in that tender place.

Finally, for those of us whose attachment figures were unnervingly inconsistent, we may discover that what arises is both an almost desperate kind of grasping and a kind of relentless inconsolability. It may seem that, no matter how much soothing and comfort a partner offers to us, it never quite reaches that place that cries out so desperately for solace. When we find in our practice that this style of preoccupied anxious ambivalence characterizes our experience of needing comfort, our practice becomes to learn to reach for and breathe into our own inconsolability, to create space for its intensity, and to begin to cultivate some small thread of faith in our basic wholeness.

Skillful Action: Seeking a Safe Harbor

We each develop our own unique vulnerabilities and fears, the places where we learn to turn away, armor up, and diminish ourselves. This becomes our place of practice as we take up the practice of intimacy.

ANCHORING BEFORE ASKING FOR SUPPORT

Learning to reach out and ask for support begins with your mindfulness meditation practice.

1. Take the experience of feeling vulnerable when needing care and, in your meditation, notice how it feels in the body. Notice the thoughts that arise

in the mind. As you notice your inconsolability, you can breathe deeply into the vividness of the experience, noticing how it flows and changes, and simply allow space for it to be present within the container of your loving awareness.

2. Anchor your attention on the breath, so that you might begin to learn that you can indeed have faith in your fundamental capacity to host even the most intense emotions. Breathe.
3. Once you have taken a moment to realize that you do not have to flee or fight with your own inner experience, you can seek the comfort of your partner's arms, receive their generosity with generosity. You can do this while not abandoning your obligation to hold your own inconsolable heart with love and spaciousness.

For the insecurely attached, this practice is learning to deny neither our vulnerable need for the care of others nor the all-too-human frailty of others. We seek care when we need it with clarity and humility, and we bow in compassionate understanding when our loved one cannot meet us there. And, in turn, we bow in endless gratitude when they can.

When the Flow Halts (No Power Position): The Perfect Storm

Even in the healthiest relationships, the attachment teeter-totter does not always flow back and forth smoothly. There will inevitably be those times when both partners are upset, reactive, and out of resources at the same time. For example, when one is in pain and the other is sick, or when both are experiencing immense stress, or when both are crushed with the intensity of a recent loss. These are moments that we often refer to as the *perfect storm*, because the elements of nature, the causes and conditions of the moment, simply happen to come together in such a way that neither partner is in any position to effectively step into the role of the secure attachment figure.

The way forward is either the path of commiseration or mutual self-care. If the emotion field is quiet and soft, like that which arises around sadness, then it may be possible to simply keep company with each other, while recognizing that both of you are out of resources. This moment actually does serve the functions of intimacy, even though in many ways you are meeting each other more from a place of equal but deep friendship.

If the emotion field is much more agitated, like that arising from irritation, frustration, and anger (but only if it's not directed at each other), then commiseration can take the form of venting together, which allows us to know that we are not alone in our frustration with the world.

Finally, however, if the hurt and anger are about the relationship, or if you simply don't have the resources for commiseration, then the wisest course in the moment is mutual self-care. For our ongoing mindfulness practice of sitting meditation, this is a particularly auspicious moment to just sit whole and upright in the open field of compassionate bare attention. Or we might check in with the physical sensations in our body, scanning with our attention our whole body from head to toe, breathing deeply, and intentionally releasing any areas of tension or discomfort. In doing so, we can release what is available to be released and then intimately allow whatever level of discomfort remains.

Again and again, in mindful attention, we are practicing coming into intimate relationship with our experience, precisely in those places where we have historically turned away from ourselves, so that we might take good and loving care of our own suffering and discomfort. As we become more and more able to do so, we may find that we suffer somewhat less, cause less damage to ourselves and others, and take better loving care of ourselves and those we care for.

The Heart of the Matter

Ultimately, the flow of the attachment system in our relationship can be cultivated as an ongoing place of intimate practice. We are called to practice with our own reactivity and vulnerability with sincerity, determination, and compassion—to seek the safe harbor when we need it. And we are called to embody the safe harbor within which our partners can weather the storms of their own being. This work will challenge our ego and soften it, if we let it, to the point where it becomes less and less a source of suffering for ourselves and others. This work will strengthen us in our capacity to meet our suffering and the suffering of others with open hearts, with great compassion, and with skillful action—for ourselves and for all beings.

Mindful Mantra

My partner is suffering.
This suffering is sacred and worthy of my full attention.
May I be a refuge and safe harbor.

I am suffering.
This suffering is sacred and worthy of my full attention.
May I seek the refuge and safe harbor of my beloved other.

My partner and I are both suffering.
Our shared suffering is sacred and worthy of my full attention.
May we each hold and harbor ourselves with loving care.
May we sit together, side by side, joined to the great earth and all beings.

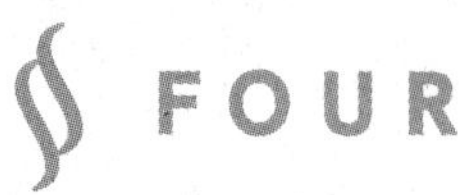

FOUR

Acting Intentionally

EVERYTHING YOU DO MATTERS

One of the most compelling findings in the relationship science literature comes out of the lab of the eminent social psychologist John Gottman at the University of Washington. In the mid-1990s, Gottman's "Love Lab" was already famous for producing some of the most persuasive and relevant research on predictors of relationship health and stability. One of the central features of John's work was that it was innovatively observational. Rather than simply using questionnaires to ask couples about their perceptions of their relationship, Gottman was convinced that the most telling signs of relationship health and deterioration were only available by observing partners while they were directly engaged in relating to each other. And so this research—and our mindfulness practice—start in the same place: with a commitment to observing the unfolding moment deeply and thoroughly.

Partners were invited into a video lab and asked to complete several questionnaires, including about common conflict areas. Once the partners identified their top areas of conflict, they were asked to spend the next 15 minutes trying to work to some resolution of that issue. Once Gottman had accumulated hundreds of recordings of couples struggling to communicate about one of their biggest areas of conflict, he and his team began the arduous work of watching all the recordings and looking for patterns that might predict how healthy those couples would end up being in the long run.

Dozens of different systems have been developed for coding and systematically observing couples' behavior. But perhaps one of the simplest and most elegant is just to observe and count the number of exchanges that are either emotionally positive or negative. In essence, this is what Gottman and his team did, with a great deal more precision and sophistication than is worth getting into here. And, though John's team found many things, one discovery that I find the most captivating is what has come to be known as the *five-to-one ratio.*

The Five-to-One Ratio

The five-to-one ratio can be thought of as the ratio of positive to negative moments between partners. To understand this in your own life, you can think of each interaction, maybe even each discernible moment of experience, between you and your partner as having a palpable emotional valence: positive, neutral, or negative. Over the course of a single interaction, a day, a week, a month, a year, and the lifetime of a relationship, those discernible moments accumulate in your mind, body, and heart in a way that becomes your fundamental felt sense of the overall emotional character of your relationship.

Stable and satisfying relationships actually require *five times* as many positive moments as negative moments.

In some ways it may seem overly simplistic, but our emotional system really is set up to perceive experiences as either pleasant or unpleasant, with things that are neither pleasant nor unpleasant registering as simply neutral. Given that, you might expect that as long as your relationship experiences an equal amount of positive interactions and negative interactions, you would feel happy and secure. However, this research has found instead that stable and satisfying relationships actually require *five times* as many positive moments as negative moments. This finding has two important implications. The first is about what we call the functioning of *P-space* and *Q-space* in the accumulation of relationship moments over time. The second is about the *impact* of negative interactions.

P-Space and Q-Space

Gottman talks about changes in relationship health occurring in two distinct spaces. In one, called P-space, change is *cumulative*. In this space, each discernible moment that occurs between you and your partner accumulates in your experience as the felt lived history of your relationship. Imagine a glass container in which all of your interactions with your partner accumulate. In this glass container, positive interactions are represented by brilliant shimmering golden balls, and negative interactions are represented by dark, cloudy gray balls. In this glass container are all of the gray and golden balls that have accumulated over the course of your *entire* relationship together. In a secure and stable relationship, the research seems to indicate that the container will have accumulated at least *five times* as many golden balls as gray balls.

Further, the research suggests that once that five-to-one ratio starts to weaken, an accumulating change in the number of gray balls starts to gradually affect our emotional sense of how safe and happy we feel in our relationship versus how anxious and unhappy we feel. As the ratio starts to fall off to four to one, three to one, and eventually one to one, our felt sense of unhappiness and distress continues to grow. The research discovered that unstable relationships (couples statistically more likely to separate or divorce) experience a ratio that is much closer to one positive for every negative interaction. And this is where it reaches a tipping point.

It is at this tipping point that we enter the realm of Q-space. Whereas P-space represents cumulative change, Q-space represents *binary* change. In this case, that binary change is our internal answer to the question, "Are you happy in your relationship?" When the container of our relationship is heavily represented by golden balls, the felt answer to the question is "Yes, I am happy in my relationship." However, at the tipping point where gray balls have become increasingly common, our answer flips to "No, I am not happy."

One of the most important points for us to take away from this research—a point that is entirely consistent with what we learn through our meditative practice—is that *every single thing that we do matters*. Every single interaction between you and your partner counts. Every positive interaction goes into the container of your relationship as a golden ball, and every negative moment goes into the container of your relationship as a gray ball—and not a single one of those balls can ever be removed. Every moment counts and is counted. And that is the first lesson of our practice in this regard. And it is why presence, attention, and mindfulness are so essential to the moment-to-moment health, well-being, and intimacy of our relationships.

The way that I envision the relationship container is that each gray ball is actually five times bigger than any one gold ball. It's the enormity of the negative encounters that knocks the wind out of us. For me, that surely fits my experience. One painful interaction between me and my partner certainly does seem to weigh so much more than it should in relation to all of the positive moments. They stay alive in my head for longer than I wish they would, and they leave me more heartsore for a longer period of time than I would want.

Inattention, thoughtlessness, and lack of care too often result in our inadvertently adding gray balls that could have otherwise been avoided. And the system is not affected by our excuses. That we were feeling tired, hungry, worn out, stressed out, grumpy, or frustrated when we stung our partner does not change a gray ball into a gold ball. It is just a gray ball, and it counts, and it can never be uncounted. This fact should sharpen our senses to the responsibility that we take on when we invite another human being into vulnerability.

Our Intention versus Our Impact

This is where it is so important for us to really understand the difference between intention and impact. Regardless of intention, it is the *impact* that accumulates here in our heart as we encounter each and all of the experiences between ourselves and our intimate other. Moments that sting get counted as gray balls in the container of our body. And this container, this warm, soft creature, is immune to our intentions. It only absorbs the impact.

When we snap at our partner, it doesn't matter that it wasn't our intention to cause harm; our partner is just harmed. When we say something that was meant to be benign or even laudatory, and it nevertheless hurts our partner's feelings, it is that impact that is counted, not our intention. When we get home later than expected, and our partner is hurt and upset, it literally does not matter that it wasn't our fault. The body counts the impact. The intention vanishes on the breeze.

It is in this spot that so many of us make a terrible mistake: We react by *defending our intentions* and inadvertently invalidate, ignore, and dismiss the *impact of our actions*. Our strong, natural instinct is toward defensiveness. In our evolutionary history, causing harm to others was the number-one reason for being expelled from the community, so we are hardwired to strongly defend any of our actions that others perceive as harmful. We say things like, "You shouldn't be upset, because I was stuck in traffic, and it wasn't my fault that I'm late." "Stop being so sensitive. Don't I get to be in a bad mood?"

The body counts the impact. The intention vanishes on the breeze.

Dismissing our harmful impact adds harm to harm. If we hurt because our partner snapped at us, and they defend their intention instead of attending to the impact, then we are hurt both by the sharpness of their sting *and* by the inadvertent (defensive) message that our hurt doesn't matter to them. Gray ball after gray ball.

In my work with couples, I see this pattern all the time. In fact, it is so common, so instinctual, that it is for all intents and purposes almost a human universal. When we see that we have harmed our partner, we defend our intent and excuse our impact. Later, if we're lucky and courageous, we might acknowledge that we caused hurt, apologize, and try to repair. But often not until we've done significantly more harm than good.

Becoming familiar with this terribly bad habit, however, not only has the potential to save us from adding gray balls to the system but might actually result in our adding several golden balls. As we've noted throughout this book, it is unavoidable that we will hurt our partner, mostly inadvertently, on a regular and ongoing basis. Hurt, vulnerability, and intimacy are intimately interwoven and of the same cloth.

A committed contemplative practice, however, can sensitize us to both our impact on others and our karmic inclination to defend ourselves at every turn. And, if we can notice when we are about to defend our intentions, we just might be able to gently guide ourselves instead to attend to our impact. And when we do *that*, we atone for and repair the harm we've caused. We strongly communicate how much we really do care when we've hurt our partner. And, once we've done *that*, once we have noticed our partner's hurt, touched it, acknowledged it, and apologized for causing it, *then* we can share our own experience of intention and circumstance. First, we might say, "I'm so sorry I'm late. I should have called the moment I realized that I was going to be. That is on me and I am so sorry. I will do better next time." Then, we might explain, "Traffic was terrible because of some accident on the freeway. I kept thinking it would clear and then it just didn't. Next time I'll call right away. I'm so sorry I worried and upset you, my love." Golden balls, golden balls, golden balls.

Really, deeply understanding the difference between intent and impact, realizing that our relational responsibility is to the impact, and vowing to practice attending to the impact first and foremost will go a long way toward keeping the ratio in our relationship weighted toward gold. But *this will take practice.* And humility. Admitting to ourselves and others that we have caused harm is being intensely vulnerable. And yet, for our purposes here, this vulnerability is at the heart of cultivating true intimacy.

Thus, in these moments when our partner tells us we have done something hurtful to them, we are given the opportunity to harness our openheartedness and our commitment to intimacy and to hold with kindness our impulse to defend our ego. Then, right there in the heart of all of that terrible discomfort, we can turn ourselves to gently tend to the harm that we have caused.

Through the practice of acknowledging our impact, we wake up to our agency and our responsibility to *great care.*

Through the practice of acknowledging our impact, we wake up to our agency and our responsibility to *great care.* What do I mean by great care? That through our interconnectedness, doing good and avoiding evil—adding golden balls and not gray balls—is always available to us. We can always assume our responsibility to take good and loving care of the unfolding moment between us and our beloved.

Setting the Intention to Accept That Everything Matters . . .

So, informed by what we know about the impact of moments that connect versus moments that wound, in keeping with the theme of this book, how might we use this knowledge in our relationships as mindfulness practice? The overall idea of the material in this book is that our relationships should

The place to start is with the practice of deeply realizing that everything we do matters, everything we do leaves its mark on our partner's heart.

ideally be a fully integrated aspect of our mindfulness practice—because, in my experience, intimate relationship is a crucible for transformation and awakening.

For me, perhaps the place to start is with the practice of deeply realizing that everything we do matters, everything we do leaves its mark on our partner's heart. This is the place where tiny details matter. And, if we're honest with ourselves, that's all there is in this life—the moment-to-moment unfolding of the specific, particular, visceral, if ephemeral, details of our lives.

From within our dedication to our practice, we vow to remain fully present, openhearted, attentive, and awake in each moment of presence with our partners—attending lovingly to our words and actions as they weave the fabric of our connection. How we pour a cup of tea. The attentiveness and spirit with which we place that cup of tea by our partner's seat. The expression we offer when we meet our partner's eye. Each act is a love letter. Each act is a manifestation of our vow to love, honor, and cherish. Having invited this beloved other into a place of vulnerability and intimacy, we care for that space, fully aware that it is sacred and precious.

Each act is a love letter.

. . . And Vowing to Respond to the Inevitability of Harm

And what of the inevitability of harm? The price of admission into intimacy is that we will regularly step on each other's toes. So we vow to be attentive to the times when we have stung our partners. We vow to accept and respond to the impact of words and actions, without rejecting their pain by defending our good and just intentions. We meet any pain we may have caused with our pain for having caused it. We bow to the moment.

We move quickly and with no hesitation to care for the harm we have caused, to soothe, reassure, and atone. And to reestablish our vow to do better in the future and to continue to learn how to take even better and better care of our partner's tender heart. In this way, we do our best to actively mend and reestablish a sense that both of us care deeply about the other's pain and well-being. I think, at the bottom, that is all that we are really seeking in those moments—some visceral sense that *our partner cares about our pain*. Even if, maybe especially if, that pain is irrational and indefensible.

None of us choose to experience being stung. It is something that comes to us unbidden. Part of our ancient, twisted karma. We need not judge it or justify it but are called simply to allow its arising openheartedly. And, from that place of holding our own pain with gentle and spacious awareness, allow ourselves to be met by our partner's concern and caring, allow ourselves to reconnect, to forgive, and to soothe in turn.

Paying Attention to What We Add to the Container

How might we actually engage in this form of practice within our intimate relationships? As always, it begins with attention. We begin with noticing the tenderness of vulnerability that characterizes a truly intimate relationship and acknowledging that we have deliberately and knowingly invited each other to step out from behind our emotional armor, promising to lovingly care for each other's defenselessness.

We also acknowledge that we remain chronically susceptible to losing our focus; to becoming self-involved, forgetful, neglectful, distracted; to letting ourselves forget our shared fragility; to relax into carelessness; to turning away from the weight of our commitment to look deeply and move with care and grace in relation to each other.

Finally, we open our hearts to the painful truth that causing each other pain and irritation is unavoidable and that we will regularly sting and irritate each other. We will hurt our partner's feelings, we will irritate them, disappoint them, and fail them. We will inadvertently push buttons that are tied to deep pools of ancient pain, and we will do this almost daily. Our partner will hurt our feelings; they will irritate, disappoint, and fail us; they will unknowingly push on our wounds, some of which may be nameless and dark to us. And our beloved will do this almost daily. And this shared tenderness is the very heart of deeply intimate relating. The only alternative is turning away, creating small pockets of hiddenness and uncaring.

NOTICING BUTTONS

We unknowingly and sometimes knowingly push our beloved's buttons. They do the same to us. They may press buttons we didn't even know we had, and vice versa. Let's explore this phenomenon.

Take out your journal and list all of your buttons, without judgment. List your tender places, the things you hold dear, along with the places that are bruised. Open up to seeing your vulnerabilities on the page. Just sit with it, noticing what comes up. Perhaps noticing an urge to leave or to "fix" what is there. Let what comes up be.

Skillful Action: Facing and Expressing Our Hurt

When, despite our intent, our impact is painful, we do not turn away from noticing. We acknowledge that we have caused pain, and we feel deeply our own pain at having done so. We apologize with sincerity. And we sincerely vow to do better. Golden balls rain down to surround and soothe the gray ball.

And what about when we ourselves have been stung?

SHARING THE STING

Again, the practice of addressing our hurt begins with attentiveness and the grounded spaciousness that we cultivate in our practice of meditation to meet with clarity the arising of pain without reaching for the cold comfort of anger or withdrawal.

1. When stung, first acknowledge that piercing, taking a moment to feel it deeply and welcome it compassionately into your experience, allowing its embodiment, breathing into its spaces, and making room for its tenderness.
2. Then turn toward your partner to tend lovingly to that tender space between you two. Discerning the appropriateness of time and space, encourage yourself to offer the gift of your *stungness*, to communicate as skillfully as you can your *ow*.

3. Invite your partner to the opportunity to catch your fall, to touch your heart, to acknowledge your ache, and to connect with caring and reassurance.
4. Together, reassure each other of your commitment to care and gentleness, honor what is vital and tremulous.

By providing this brief moment of pause and connection, you can then reengage together the various demands of the day.

We do this over and over, taking up each moment in its freshness without hesitation or fatigue. As has been said by Thich Nhat Hanh, when the left hand is hurt, the right hand just reaches to care for it, and the left hand leans into that caring. This is the practice of vow and repent.

When we have been stung, we enter into the spiritual crucible of intimacy. We are called to alchemize our ancient wounds, to heal the places where we are easily hurt, to attend lovingly to our vulnerabilities as we cultivate equanimity and compassion. We both seek out the care of our partner and (perhaps more importantly) turn inward to attend lovingly and responsibly to the places where we are hooked.

Rather than focusing on our partner as the cause, if we can meet our pain as *our* pain, which has been given into *our* care, then we can not only care for ourselves, but we can also begin the practice of transforming our pain into wisdom. We can practice holding our vulnerabilities with tenderness and recognize that there is an inherent strength in vulnerability, that who and what we are need not shrink from connection, that we can handle our own vulnerability without turning away from ourself, from our partner, or from the world.

You can begin the practice of transforming your pain into wisdom.

The relationship caution here is that, when gray balls are not attended to with conscientiousness and care, they can metastasize, growing in toxicity and resentment into painful masses of separation, avoidance, and a kind of soreness that is easily retriggered. Nothing swept under the rug ever really stays there. This is the *truly intimate* practice of relationship. We turn toward these places as a practice of intimacy, connection, and interwovenness, acknowledging our fundamental interconnectedness as we co-create the exquisite vividness of a living dynamic relationship.

Just as important—or, rather, five times as important—we turn to the role of practice-honed attention on the accumulation of gold balls. Thich Nhat Hanh regularly reminds us that love is not so much a feeling as it is an act of skillfulness.

ACCUMULATING GOLD BALLS

From that place where attention is the most basic form of love, commit yourself to the lifelong practice of learning what your partner needs from you moment to moment to feel cared for, honored, and treasured.

Commit yourself to the privilege of artfully loving your partner with, perhaps:

- A cup of coffee
- A soft touch
- A sweet note
- A playful flirt
- A long walk
- A listening ear
- A soft place to land at the end of a long day in the hard world
- Or anything that meets their need to feel loved

As each of us is always becoming and becoming, so too are our partners, in each day and each moment, arriving into our lives as new and undiscovered beings. We attend and learn and care, not falling into habits of inattentiveness, certainty, and carelessness. So, for us, in this practice of true intimacy, we carry with us this living question: "How do I best love you today, my dear?"

The Heart of the Matter

First, we recognize that all things we do and fail to do matter, and we set the intention to take advantage of every opportunity to deliberately place golden balls into the container. We practice waking up from distraction and preoccupation over and over again so that we might say or do something kind, celebrate successes both big and small, provide encouragement and loving support, engage with affection and sensuality, and in any other way possible become a source of love and joy in our partner's life.

Second, with mindful attention, we practice noticing when we have hurt our partner, and we turn toward them, acknowledge their pain, apologize, soothe, and vow to do better. Read Chapter 12 to learn more about the practice of forgiveness and repair and to better practice surrounding gray balls with the golden balls of repair.

Then, when we ourselves experience hurt, with mindful attention, we turn toward our hurt, acknowledge it, hold it gently and with great self-compassion with our attention until we are able to skillfully communicate our pain with kindness to our partner so that they might care and repair.

Finally, we practice, each of us, taking personal responsibility for the state of the magic ratio in our relationship, not pawning that responsibility off on to our partner but, instead, wholly owning that right now, in this very moment. Tell yourself, "I can start adding golden balls and repairing gray balls. My relationship is *my* relationship. I vow to make it shine."

Mindful Mantra

May I see you and know your tenderness.
May I always care for you with love.
May I honor both your fragility and strength, our connectedness and your independence, and our shared commitment to vulnerability and authenticity.
May I acknowledge and tend to any pain that I cause you, and may I offer any pain that I may experience into your loving care.
May I make it my lifelong practice to fill our space with an abundance of love and joy.

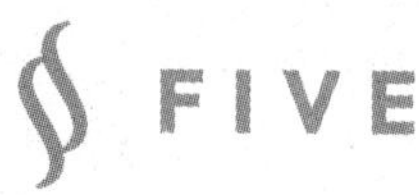

FIVE

Listening Deeply

MAY I ONLY SEEK TO UNDERSTAND

Listen.
Just for a moment.

Stop what you are doing, sit back, and just let the sounds of the moment enter your ears. Don't reach for them. Just let them come. Receive the sounds of the world in this moment without comment or complaint. If you can, let your sense of a separate self drop away and allow yourself to be nothing other than hearing what is happening. Rest in this pure hearing.

Deep listening is an intimacy practice. It requires deliberately bringing forth our full attention and cultivating a willingness to receive whatever is offered as a gift, graciously received, without judgment, and without critical commentary.

Selective Hearing

Too often we do not listen to truly understand and empathize. Instead, we listen only to react and respond. We listen only until we have something to say, then we stop listening until we get an opportunity to say it. Instead of listening to the other, we listen only to ourselves, holding our attention on what we want to say while the other person's talking plays unheeded in the background. We listen only until the other person says something that we can comment on, react to, or refute.

I see this often in working with couples in therapy. It unfolds like this: One partner will say something that makes the other partner feel mischaracterized or described unfairly, and then nothing else registers for that partner until they have an opportunity to defend themselves. Consider Sophia and Alex.

> In session, Sophia described how Alex came down the stairs and angrily kicked one of the kids' toys across the room, then walked into the kitchen grumbling. She said, "I just don't know why he has to start the day off in such a cranky mood." Sophia admits that we all get up on the wrong side of the bed, but it's upsetting, and she feels like it's happening more frequently lately. She gives another example of his coming home from work in a similarly grumpy mood, not really greeting her, and just going off to the living room to sullenly watch TV. She says she tried to ask him about his day, and he just snapped that he didn't want to talk about it.
>
> After some reflection and acknowledgment, I turn to Alex. I note that Sophia genuinely cares about his upset, even as it is simultaneously difficult to meet it, and ask him how it is for him when Sophia is grumpy. Alex orients and looks at me and says, "I didn't angrily kick Timmy's truck across the room. I tripped over it and twisted my ankle, and that's why she thought I was so grumpy."

And there it is. Nothing past the truck got in.

If we're honest with ourselves, it is often like this. We get caught by something our partner said, and we just cannot keep listening until we can say our thing. It doesn't even have to be something unpleasant. It can just be that we remembered something else we wanted to share, a story we wanted to tell, or a point we wanted to make. Our hearing goes in and out, catching bits and pieces, but mostly we are lost in our own thoughts, afraid that if we let our thing go, we'll never get it back. We're more concerned with ourselves than with the other.

In some ways that is the heart of it: being more concerned with ourselves than with our partner. As though, if we were to give ourselves over to only listening to understand, we might lose hold of ourselves, be forgotten, not listened to, not cared about. If I listen to you, then what about me?

Setting the Intention to Be a Better Listener

Deep listening is a radically selfless act. We gift ourselves the opportunity to put our self-concern aside for a moment, to let go of our own need to be propped up, tended to, seen, heard, and reassured that we exist. We take advantage of the opportunity to care more about understanding than about being understood, to care more in this moment about our beloved's perspective than our own, to lower the barrier between self and other, so that we can just be this resonance. This is the practice of true intimacy.

Here are some simple things to keep in mind. First, simply notice and accept that *not listening* is our natural state. Our attention is most often on our inner monologue, our worries, or our habitual distractions—thinking about dinner, work, a conversation with a friend, chores, the latest TV show we saw, how we are feeling, a problem that needs to be solved. Up our own asses, as it were. This is fine. Not a problem. The human condition.

Deep listening is a radically selfless act.

The second thing to know and keep in mind is that true listening is more active than passive. Simply put, listening is something that we *do*, on purpose, with intention, and it requires a determination to exert the energy necessary to sustain attention and actively hold open our receptivity. If we are not actively sustaining our attention, it is quite naturally of the nature to wander.

Finally, our ongoing meditation practice provides us with plenty of opportunity to notice that self-concern is the biggest barrier. The more we are thinking about ourselves—what we want, what we need, what we have to say, what the impact is on us, what the implication of what we're hearing is for us, how what we're hearing affects the self-narrative that we are so invested in protecting—the less available we are to listen deeply for the sake of empathy, compassion, understanding, and true intimacy.

Of course, this doesn't mean that we make ourselves available for abuse or that we let ourselves be harmed or treated disrespectfully. Our concern for our own well-being is also the enactment of compassion. However, when are fully engaged in the act of intimate listening, our primary concern must be thoroughly understanding the other from within their own flesh and bones. Taking up how our partner's views and perspectives affect us is a concern for another time, *after* we have heard and understood.

So that's it. Intimate listening is not our natural state, it takes effort and attention, and we must put our own ego aside to be truly open. Easy, right?

If only it were so. . . .

Paying Attention to the Present While Listening

The practice of deep listening begins with gently ushering our attention into this moment, anchoring our present-moment attention in our ears and in the part of our mind that can imagine ourselves in our partner's shoes. Again, as in any mindfulness practice, our capacity to stay present-centered and attentive can be nurtured and developed with intentional practice. We set the intention to not let our attention wander, and, when it does, to bring it back to deep listening as quickly and as often as possible. Wash, rinse, repeat. Attend, return, repeat. As a reminder, see Chapter 1 for ways to practice mindful attention.

Skillful Action: Learning to Listen Deeply

To put this into practice, we must deliberately put aside our own self-concern for the time being. For this moment of listening and receiving, it isn't about us. It's about understanding our partner's perspective, thoughts, feelings, and views as thoroughly and empathically as possible. Our goal in this moment is to understand both intellectually and emotionally; to understand what our partner is thinking and to feel what our partner is feeling. We call this *compassionate understanding.*

Then we activate and use the part of our mind that can imagine what it is like to be thoroughly within our partner's perspective. We call to mind what we know about their life; we imagine what it is like to think their thoughts and how those thoughts arise out of how they genuinely perceive the world. We allow ourselves to feel their feelings as our own, with no separation. We call this practice *empathic imagination*. The use of our empathic imagination as the basis for not just listening, but *deep* listening, is the primary method of cultivating truly compassionate understanding.

This can be an intensely vulnerable and challenging practice. There is a part of us that doesn't even want to feel our own feelings, much less intimately experience the emotions of someone, anyone, else—maybe especially the one we are closest to and whose suffering touches us the most deeply and who has stung us the most frequently. That history of stinging and being stung can make it especially hard for us to open our hearts fully to receive our partner's pain, or even joy, completely and without pushing some part of it away.

Our ego, our self-concern, our own hurt can strongly resist allowing ourselves to intimately and compassionately understand. I think this is why it is sometimes, maybe even often, so much easier to empathize with and compassionately understand a stranger, acquaintance, or friend than our own partner. There is just so much less at stake, fewer of our own feelings on the line, and fewer implications for our own wants and preferences with a stranger.

So deep listening becomes the opportunity for the real practice of meeting the arising of our ego defenses and hosting them with great care and spaciousness, so that we might continue the much more selfless work of truly intimate compassionate understanding.

What If Our Partner Is Saying Something We Don't Want to Hear?

A significant part of the challenge is that our partner will say things that we don't want to hear, that we don't like hearing, and that we will have a reaction to. We must make room for those arisings, host them with compassion and spaciousness, and keep listening. We need to continue to prioritize feeling our way into our partner's experience, holding ourself, our heart, and our ears open.

This is the difficult spiritual work of not letting your ego always have its way. It's okay to feel stung, to notice defensiveness arising, to feel misperceived and misunderstood. Receive all of that with boundless care while continuing to breathe, let go, and hold your focus on listening to understand compassionately. Remember, a true spiritual practice plays rough with the ego, and this is a true spiritual practice.

Once we have begun to genuinely, empathically, and compassionately understand, it is essential that we communicate that understanding to our partner. So much of what we are yearning for from each other is to have the experience of being empathized with, compassionately understood, known, and accepted. We just want to feel that someone else, especially our intimate partner, really understands what it's like to be us—from the inside, accepting and holding our experience as real, truly present, and validly experienced. I continue to be strongly convinced that all the joys of relationship flow from cultivating heartfelt empathy and that all the suffering and sorrows of relationship flow from its lack.

Putting Our Understanding into Words

So we put our understanding into words. We might say, "My love, I can feel that you are sad and scared and that your mind is so worried about the implications and what might happen if I take this job. I get all of that. And of course you feel that way. Of course." To a degree, the more details we can include in our reflection, the more deeply understood our partner will feel. And the more deeply understood they feel, the closer and more intimate our relationship becomes in that moment, as we actively lower the barrier between self and other—another gold ball in the container.

Sometimes, at this point our understanding is still not complete and true. So we invite our partner to help correct or tailor any part of our understanding that may still be out of alignment with their experience.

> ***Correction:*** "I don't know, I guess it's not really that I'm worried about what might happen. It's more that I'm feeling sad about how it has already turned out."
>
> ***Response to correction:*** "Yeah, I can feel that. . . . It is sad; it makes sense to feel the depth of that sadness."

Again, having our empathic reflection corrected may be an ego-challenging experience, but the practice is to gratefully accept any correction, to weave that correction into our understanding, and to try again to share what we have come to know of our partner's inner world. And, when we do, when we really get it, this is everything.

This is everything. Another gold ball.

Avoid Jumping to Problem Solving

It is important to hold this moment of understanding without fixing anything or problem solving. Jumping too quickly into problem solving can be a kind of turning away that diminishes the intimacy and connection of the moment. We problem-solve to escape. That's a good thing. And shared problem solving can itself be intimate. Still, for a breath or two, simply bask in this moment of shared understanding. It is enough. And more often than you might think, it is everything.

Now, if you must, and if it is wise, rooted in this place of deep understanding, you can begin to take action toward problem solving. If there are things to do that would be helpful, do them. And have faith that when you act from a place of true empathy, your actions are much more likely to be skillful and beneficent—to do more good than harm.

THE PATH TO DEEP LISTENING

Arriving at deep listening is not a straight line on a map. But if engaged with intention, compassion, and awareness, you can arrive.

1. Lower your ego flag.
2. Set your intention on cultivating compassionate understanding.
3. Center your attention on the part of your mind that listens.
4. Activate your empathic imagination.
5. Breathe through your reactivity and stay committed to deep understanding.
6. Communicate your compassionate understanding clearly.
7. Accept correction.
8. Give the moment of intimate connection time to breathe.
9. When necessary, act with wisdom and skill.

The capacity to stay mindfully present and the capacity to wake up and notice when we are distracted and preoccupied grows with our ongoing dedicated meditation practice. In other words, the capacity to mindfully attend and listen deeply isn't just something that we force with our willpower. It is instead a growing predilection to an attentive state that we slowly build and nurture through our regular meditation practice.

As we practice returning our attention to the present moment again and again through, for example, meditation on the breath, we become more frequently mindfully and attentively present. As we become more frequently mindfully and attentively present, we are increasingly able to pull ourselves out of our distracted state and to purposefully focus on what our partner is saying. Our heart becomes more resonant as we practice empathically imagining their experience, and our responses become more genuine and caring.

Just as we practice bringing our attention back to breath during our meditation practice, we similarly practice bringing our attention back to our partner's voice, presence, and meaning. We practice noticing and letting go of our preoccupation with our own concerns, so that we can attend fully to our partner's experience. We practice this interconnectedness over and over again. A lifetime of ongoing practice. And, if we're lucky, we realize for ourselves that we are not separate by even a hair's breadth. We awaken from the dream of separation to know a depth of true intimacy that is clear, boundless, and ever flowing.

We awaken from the dream of separation to know a depth of true intimacy that is clear, boundless, and ever flowing.

The Heart of the Matter

The practice of deep listening leads to awakening. As we practice giving ourselves completely to the mission of thoroughly and compassionately understanding the experience of another human being—our beloved partner—we come to realize that we are all pieces of the same whole. As we practice putting aside our own concerns and reactivity so that we might know our partner ever more deeply, intimacy flourishes.

Mindful Mantra

My partner calls out to me, through words and silence.
May I hear with both ears and heart.
May I listen deeply.

May I resonate with my whole being.
May I drop all barriers that come between us.
May I put myself aside so that I might bear full witness.
May the boundary of self and other drop away that we might together be blessed with true intimacy.
Your joy is my joy. Your pain is my pain.
In the sea of nonseparation, there is only love.

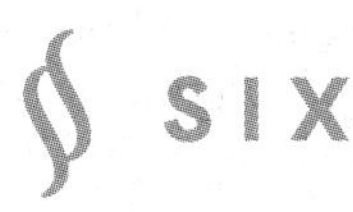

SIX

Waking Up to Interconnectedness

THE ILLUSION OF SEPARATENESS

Zen master Thich Nhat Hanh, in his singularly pithy and precise way, points right to the heart of the matter when he says, "We are here to awaken from the illusion of separateness." The whole point of our existence, the meaning of life, as it were, is to wake up from our trance-like conviction that we are separate from and alone in the universe. We are here to remember and experience our interwovenness with each other and with all things. Though we believe that we are alone, we are, in fact, innumerable.

Though our interconnectedness is one of the most fundamental truths of existence, an embodied awareness of that fact can be difficult to achieve and rare to experience. The promise, however, is that waking up to our fundamentally interdependent nature ultimately relieves a great deal of our unnecessary suffering. Almost all contemplative traditions include this recognition as an aspiration of the practice. Oneness with God, the great earth, the universe, or all beings. True intimacy is not separate.

True intimacy is realizing our nonseparateness from all things, but especially from each other.

True intimacy is realizing our nonseparateness from all things, but especially from each other.

THE LONELY DREAM

Aaron and Kelly have been together for 20 years, having met and fallen in love in college when they were paired to put a presentation together for their psychology seminar. Over the years, they've had two children and have wholly taken up the life of family and careers. Aaron is a salesman, and Kelly is an oncologist. They live a life of "divide and conquer" to manage all the many demands on their time. Kelly gets the kids ready for school in the morning, and Aaron manages the evenings of chores, sports, and homework. They share responsibility for the upkeep of the house, each having fallen into their separate domains. Kelly does the bills. Aaron takes care of the yard. Kelly shops for groceries. Aaron makes most of the meals. Laundry, cleaning, repairs, chauffeuring, scheduling are juggled in chaos, but somehow it all works and they manage to keep their heads above water—mostly.

And yet they are both not just stressed but lonely. Surrounded by family, friends, and colleagues, maybe each in their own way, and still. . . . more alone than either of them has ever been. In the quiet moments—walking to the car after work, loading laundry in the basement, mowing endless rows in the lawn—it hits them, weighing them each down with that subtle ache, "Why do I feel so overwhelmed and so lonely?"

Look, everything we do, everything we say, everything we think, every breath we take affects our partner. Though we may imagine it otherwise, we are not separate by even a hair's breadth. The air we breathe out, they breathe in. The path we forge, they follow. The dish we wash, they eat from. The anger we harbor, they moor in. Maybe we wish that it were otherwise. It isn't.

The practice of awakening, of wakefulness, of mindfulness and awareness, is to recognize, realize, and hold this truth in mind, to feel the truth of it in our body, in every moment of our day. For example, here I am, typing at my computer; this both affects and is affected by my partner. I stop clicking the keys and sigh, she looks over, glances at my computer screen, reads the last sentence I wrote, smiles, and asks how it's going. We talk for a moment, and then it takes her a minute to reorient to what she was doing, and I give her hand a little

Everything we do, everything we say, everything we think, every breath we take affects our partner.

squeeze of encouragement. We both continue typing. The gates are open; the borders are porous; giver, receiver, and gift are not separate. Life and death, we are interwoven.

This experience of interconnectedness, of dependent co-arising, that we co-create each other, is antithetical to what we have been conditioned to believe and experience. Especially in an individualistic culture, but even so in more collectivist cultures, we believe in and experience our separateness. This is our habit of mind: *I wash this dish to have a clean dish and put it away in the cupboard, and that's it. It all happens in my own little narcissistic cocoon, and if it affects anyone else, well, that's their problem. This dish I fail to wash, leaving it on the counter (for now), with the remnants of last night's spaghetti on it, is my choice alone.* Though we can't help knowing that others will see this dirty plate throughout the day, we let that knowing get fuzzy, out of focus, obscuring any available clarity about the unavoidable and ongoing impact of our action on others. We collude with our own blinding. Mute our own knowing. Sever and turn away from our true intimacy.

That is the illusion of separation. Our own private hell of disconnection.

Setting the Intention to Breathe Each Other into Being

So what is the actual truth of nonseparation? And, even more importantly, how do we practice it? The truth of the matter, what we discover when we examine our experience deeply, minutely, and unflinchingly, is that we are ceaselessly co-creating each other. We breathe each other into being. In Buddhism, the term used to point to this phenomenological truth is dependent *co-arising*. Or, as Thich Nhat Hanh states it, *interdependence*. Put most simply, this means that who you are in this moment is an open medley of all the things that are happening in and around you at this moment, from the community of flora living out lifetimes in your gut to the complexity of geopolitical transnational relations. And who you are in this moment is unfailingly woven out of your relationships and how you have been shaped by them. As the ingredients in that vast medley change, so do you. And as you change, so does your partner.

As soon as you meet, you start the process of co-creating each other. Your eyes meet, she smiles, and you are forever changed. You share something true, he touches your hand, and you are rebuilt. And, as the moments accumulate and the days, weeks, and years go by, you give birth together to endless co-created moments, whole languages arise and fall between you, your skin and cells intermingle, and you are transformed—again and again.

All of this happens and is true and inexorable and incessant, regardless of whether you are aware of it or not. It is simply the truth of the matter. And though intimacy is our natural state, we cannot know this and be made whole by it until we are awake to it, see and experience it with clear and acute awareness. We must wake up to our union. And to do this, we must practice.

Paying Attention to Your Partner's Presence

So what might this practice consist of? How do we do this? Well, first, as in all awakening practices, it starts with attention and awareness. When our partner comes into the room, notice how that changes us. How their presence has undeniable impact. How their presence changes everything. When they leave the room, again, notice how the sensations in our body shift, how the states and contours of our mind and heart take a slightly different shape. Use both lovingly curious observation and empathic imagination to try to get a feel for how our partner is influenced, shaped, and changed when we enter and when we leave. Notice how our presence has undeniable impact. How our presence changes everything.

We can learn a lot about what we have co-created by engaging in this simple exercise. With this practice of awareness, perhaps we might find ourselves being more mindful and more conscientious about the ingredients that we bring to the mix. Our tone of voice, the quality of our gaze, the softness of our gestures, the language of our bodies. When we sit next to our partner, on the couch, at the table, in the car, notice the quality of the air, the atmosphere, how our body feels, what arises in our mind, how the emotional mist shifts and swirls. Notice and imagine how body, mind, and heart might be shifting for this other human being at our side. Practice being awake to all of it, moment to arising moment. Anchor our attention to the feel of our partner's presence in our body, mind, and heart, as well as the feel of our partner's experience of *our* presence on their body, mind, and heart. Feel in your bones the experience of how you are co-creating each other, moment after moment, breath after breath.

Know your role and responsibility in this. This is how we practice intimacy. We blend the ingredients of our being. It has always been so.

If we choose to take this up as a practice, we will find that it is available to us in every moment, as reliable as our breath, whether we are physically with our partner or not. When we are not with them, we bring them to mind—we notice how our internal landscape changes. How what we are wanting and not wanting arise differently. How the quality of mind and heart that we nurture and cultivate affects the quality of the mix.

When we are together with our partner, we pay attention, as much as possible, on a moment-to-moment basis, feeling for the texture and tasting the flavor of this moment being co-created, without judgment, just noticing and holding it as clearly as we can. As with the breath practice, we need to notice when our attention wanders away to other things and then gently shepherd it back to awareness of the many qualities of the moment being co-created. Words are not necessary. See how our deepening experience of interconnectedness, just by itself, adds new and different flavors to the mix.

We bring our curiosity to this practice. We pay close attention to the types of ingredients we are adding to the soup of the shared body, then sip a spoonful and really taste it. Are we adding bitter herbs, with our tone, with our words, or even with the thoughts that we are muttering to ourselves, over and over again, in the privacy of our own skull? What are the attitudes that we are cultivating in our heart? What flavor do they add? What happens when we add dollops of sweetness? Or, what about when we drop in something savory, sensuous, and rich? Blending and blending. Noticing and noticing.

As we open ourself to this experience, to feeling the truth of it in your flesh, it can be an intensely vulnerable experience, and maybe even a little overwhelming. We are so habitually used to shielding ourselves from knowing this truth, and we are in many ways so comforted inside the hard shell of our separation, that lowering those defenses, even for a brief period of silent practice, can feel threatening and overexposed. Please, if you can, breathe into this vibrant tremor, make room for it, allow it to pass over and through you, remind yourself that you are safe and in actuality no more exposed than you ever are—just more aware of it—more intimate.

Skillful Action: Co-Creating Your Existence

This simple act of mindful noticing is transformative. Let's lay out the steps to practice co-creating in a simpler fashion.

STEPS TO CO-CREATION

1. **Gently gather your attention to the present moment:** When in your partner's presence, just like with the breath meditation, simply notice what arises naturally, without trying to change anything, simply observing the quality of your shared experience. What is that like? To feel for the subtle and maybe not so subtle moment-by-moment shifts in the tone and tenor of the music your relationship makes, as you breathe in and they breathe out. As you tap your foot and they scratch their head. As they sip their coffee and you scroll on your phone. Remain mindful of the ongoing flow of interrelationship, with boundless acceptance.
2. **Bring your partner into your circle of awareness:** Widen your attention to palpably include your partner. As you breathe in and out, anchor your attention in the flow of your experience of your partner's presence. Tune into and embody the moment-to-moment, continuous unfolding of your co-creation. Allow yourself to simply receive and savor the changes as you experience them in your body, heart, and mind.
3. **Notice what you are adding to the moment:** Draw your attention to what you are adding to the mix that affects the melody. What bodily experiences are you bringing? What tensions, tightness, constrictions? What calm, ease, affection? What thoughts are arising in your mind? What sentences? Are they bitter or sweet? What attitudes are you holding—embracing or rejecting? Can you feel a difference between when you are mindfully attuned to your duet and when you are hypnotized into one of the many trances of separation and self-involvement? Just notice.
4. **Notice how you are affected:** Begin to notice how, like stones dropped in a pond, every sight, sound, or sensation that you receive from your partner creates ripples in your being. Notice how every moment of unfolding affects and changes you. Hold yourself open to this change. Allow it. Gratefully receive it. Surrender to it. Notice with kindness how you might try to protect yourself from this vulnerability and encourage yourself to stay open. Then return your attention to noticing how everything your partner does, says, and feels causes a shift in your experience, in your

body, in your mind, and in your heart. Every sigh, every swallow, every flicker of a finger or toe resonates.

5. **Tune into the experience of interwovenness:** Bring your attention not just to how your partner is actively creating both of you in this moment, but also to how your *reception* of the ingredients they are adding strongly affects the flavor of your co-creation. Feeling even more deeply, notice how you cannot help vividly experiencing your partner's feelings. How their emotional state blends intimately with your emotional state. How is it for you in your body and mind when they are sad? When they are irritated? When they are happy? When they are anxious? When they are feeling loved and safe? Notice how you are receiving your partner. When your partner is sad, notice how the resonance of the moment changes when you are open to and make room for that sadness and how it changes when you resist and reject that sadness. Are you receiving your partner with openheartedness, gratitude, acceptance, generosity, and grace? Or are you receiving your partner with judgment, rejection, and bitterness? Try to practice receiving what is arising as sacred, as the path of liberation itself. Acknowledge the experience of interwovenness. There is no separation between you and your partner. This endlessly unfolding moment is just thus. Intimacy.

Here's an example:

Step 1: Mel gets home from the grocery store, and Kris brings her full attention to Mel's arrival. She pauses, breathes, and notices how her shoulders just naturally relax knowing that Mel is home safe and sound.

Step 2: Kris asks Mel how the store was, and as they unpack the groceries they start talking about their day. Kris attunes deeply to the nuanced changes in her experience as she and Mel interact and connect. She notices the rhythm in which they do the grocery dance, Mel putting away the cereal and canned beans in the pantry, herself focused on the fruits and vegetables in the fridge. In this recognition she smiles—thinking of all the times they have put groceries away together, all the little bumps, sighs, and "You're standing right where I need to be"s they had to navigate to find this much more graceful dance.

Step 3: Kris starts to draw her attention to what she is bringing to the moment. She feels the impulse to jump in and be the first to share about her day. She notices that she has a somewhat agitated energy that is arising from the thought that "I have too many things to do and too little time to do them in." She listens to the tone of her voice when she asks about Mel's day—mindful to be genuine and curious rather than rote and monotonous. She notices that some part of her mind continues to be distracted by work and the kids and the clock getting ever closer to the dog's dinner time.

Step 4: In her practice of expanding her attention to how Mel is affecting her experience, Kris notices that, at least in this moment, she feels comforted and eased by Mel's presence. She sees Mel's inquisitive glance, checking in to see how she's feeling, and she hears herself offer an audible sigh, recognizing that everything that needs to get done will be easier now that they are both home. She recognizes that some concern arises when Mel gets a small crease between the eyes talking about work deadlines. This brings up some worry about finances and how they are going to make it if Mel decides to look for another job, potentially leading to a period of time with only one income. She feels the intensity of this thought tugging her away from the moment and away from what Mel is actually saying about work. With grace she recognizes that money is one of her most significant buttons and that when her thoughts wander to money, she has a difficult time not going straight to problem-solving mode. With compassion she brings herself back to the moment. Allowing all of it to just be here as the unfolding of MelKris.

Step 5: Kris primarily notices that she is receiving the moment by feeling both the relief of Mel's presence and the added concern about jobs and finances. She admits that she wishes that Mel was happier at work. She also notices her judgment that Mel often complains about deadlines but very rarely makes changes to meet them earlier. This judgment is followed by the recognition that they are both doing their best and contributing to their family in important ways. She sets the intention to receive the complexity of the moment with an open heart and compassionate presence. She lets her body feel the unfolding of the moment, just as it is. As they finish the grocery waltz, they transition into the dinner tango.

Integration Into Daily Life

The practice as described above can be taken up as a formal practice, in which we sit with stillness and intention for a dedicated period of time, practicing mindfulness of all the dimensions of dependent co-arising. It can also be of profound benefit to ourselves and to our relationships to practice integrating this quality of awareness into our day-to-day lives. When the alarm goes off and we wake together, rather than knitting the container of the separate self closed, we can practice opening our awareness fully to our partner's presence and allowing ourselves to be drawn into being and into wakefulness.

We can set our intention to practice our clear awareness of nonseparation whenever we are together in the same space. Brushing our teeth. Dancing each other through the swirl of our morning routine. Meeting our moment of parting for the day with reverence and love. Holding our partner mindfully in our hearts from time to time throughout the day. Entering the moment of greeting each other at the end of the day by fully arriving with our whole being and taking a few dedicated moments to savor our connection. Giving ourselves to the practice of creating our evening together with dedication, awareness, and presence. Resting in the faithfulness of how our partner, and the universe, sings us into being.

Importantly, we must take it easy on ourself. This practice is a lot to take in. As I've said before, intimacy is not for the faint of heart. And yet we need not carry this practice of concentrated attention relentlessly. Our natural state will reassert itself, and we can rest there when we need to. We can pick up the practice for a period. Throw ourselves into it as if our life depends on it. We can journal about the experience, then put it down when we need to and resume our normal programming. Stepping forward and stepping back, we will grow in our ability to stay attuned to our present-moment interconnectedness.

And, as in all of this practice of inter-being, we notice the beneficial effects of mindful speech and the often painful effects of mindless speech. Knowing that every word that leaves our mouth changes our partner, and that change cannot be undone. We vow to take up the practice of mindful speech with unwavering respect for the power of our words. We commit to taking responsibility for our every utterance. And, in doing so, we do our best to speak with great care and a loving heart. Regardless of whether we are talking about something easy or hard, we touch deeply our interconnectedness, we call up our empathy and connection of heart, and from that place of tenderness, we choose our words with care.

The Heart of the Matter

We inherit the illusion of separateness. We bring this conviction that we are separate into our relationships. We are strongly inclined to create and defend the construction of the separate self in the service of our small ego. We believe that we *are* our ego and that, if it is shiny and accomplished and worthy of praise by others, then we might be accepted and loved. But, if it is denigrated, sullied, criticized, or judged, we will be diminished and rejected. And then we constrict.

When we constrict, we become more seemingly isolated, beset, and alone. Though it is inescapable, we are convinced that what we do doesn't affect, or at least doesn't *always* affect, our partner. Yet, everything that we do and say and everything that we fail to do or say affects our partner (and all beings). Likewise, everything our partner does and says and everything that our partner fails to do or say affects us (and all beings). We can practice the exquisite intimacy of each moment of our co-creation. And, through this practice, we can awaken from the dark dream of separation.

Mindful Mantra

As I enter into your presence, may I know that we are not separate.
May I feel your breath as my breath,
your heart as my heart,
my wounds as your wounds,
my hopes as your hopes,
my joys as your joys.
May I never forget the power of my words and actions on your tender heart.
May I remain open to the power of your words and actions on my tender heart.
May we practice together building this sacred cairn, stone by faithful stone, so that we and all beings might know love and liberation.

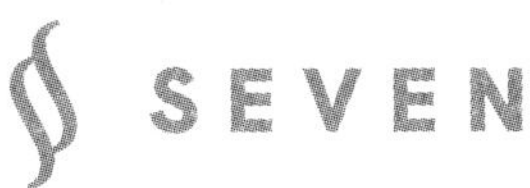

SEVEN

Loving Your Partner Skillfully

MAY YOU KNOW THAT I ADORE YOU

We most commonly think about love as an emotion, but in this chapter I am going to invite you to begin cultivating love as a practice—both a relational and a spiritual practice. Love as a spiritual practice serves to get us out of our own way, to soften the hard shell of our self-concern, so that we might free ourselves from suffering and awaken from the illusion of separateness. We want to take love from a feeling into a daily practice of skillful action. We want to take up this practice with intention, determination, and perhaps, if we have any sense of what we are getting into, at least a small quiver of trepidation.

Usually, we use the word *love* to mean our experience of some combination of affection, attachment, and yearning. To say "I love you" in an intimate relationship can be akin to saying something like "I crave you" or "I am fond of you" or even "I am committed to you." This, in and of itself, is really quite wonderful. I express my felt experience of affection, attraction, commitment, fondness, admiration, and yearning by saying "I love you."

We can learn, through careful attention and practice, how to be even more artfully loving.

That said, from the perspective of relationship as a spiritual practice, we want to grow beyond cultivating a deeper and deeper affection for our partner (and a widening circle of affection for others). We also want to attend closely to the fact that our love can be enacted in ways that are more or less skillful. We want to begin to notice that how we enact our love can sometimes do more harm than good—or at least not do as much good as we would like. We want to begin to know for ourselves that we can learn, through careful attention and practice, how to be even more artfully loving.

Unskillful Love

Unskillful love commonly shows up in couples when one partner is seeking emotional support and the other partner offers problem-solving support instead (or vice versa).

> Jess came home from work and started to complain about a colleague, just wanting to vent and get some commiseration. Jess had had some uncomfortable interactions with the colleague before and was seeking some empathy and understanding from her partner. Charlie could see that Jess was upset. He wanted to help her feel better, so he racked his brain for the best possible solution. So he offered, "Well, have you tried. . . . ?" Unfortunately, for Jess, his response felt meddlesome, and even a little condescending, and definitely didn't feel like the commiseration that she was seeking. So she replied, "What? It's not even about that. . . ." Their conversation ended in a little tiff, with Jess feeling unsupported and Charlie feeling rejected, upset, and confused. To Charlie, problem solving is exactly what he would have been looking for if he were the one who was complaining.

Another quick example from closer to home. My love does not have much of a sweet tooth. In fact, she really hates things that are too sweet. Her mother, on the other hand, has quite a well-developed sweet tooth. For her mother, the sweeter the better. When her mom is visiting, and she sees that her daughter is particularly stressed, and she wants to care for her and bring her a little bit of joy, she buys cookies and cakes and brings her very sweet coffee. It is so clear that all of this is a mother's affection for and attempt to do something loving for her daughter. And yet. My love does not have much of a sweet tooth. Over the years, my partner's mom has learned that skillful gestures of love for her daughter are more likely to involve fruit and jasmine tea. For all of us, the hope lies in the fact that once we know better, we can do better.

We try to love our partners in our way, rather than learning how to love them in their way. If we're honest with ourselves, we might begin to notice that this is not uncommon. Sometimes the people around us, from a place of genuine affection, care, and commitment, do or say things that hurt us, disappoint us, or make us suffer. Equally, sometimes, from a place of genuine affection, care, and commitment, we do and say things that cause the people we love to suffer.

I want to suggest that we do this because we are actually thinking more about ourselves than about the person we love. In these moments, we are operating from a place of separateness, seeing our partner through the lens of our own self-absorption, encased in our own ego bubble, and therefore fundamentally out of touch with the uniqueness of our partner and thus insensitive to how best to care for them so that they might thrive and be happy. The vow to care for our partner as ourselves is at the heart of a spiritual practice. In the previous chapter, we learned that everything we say and do has an impact on our beloved. Everything our beloved says and does has an impact on us. Everything we don't say and fail to do has an impact on our love. Everything our love doesn't say and fails to do has an impact on us. We practice toward embodying nonseparation and seeing through the film of ego that blocks us from true intimacy.

Consider how we might learn to care for a new plant. Let's say the person I love the most in the world gave me a beautiful flowering plant—one I've never seen or taken care of before. I immediately fall madly in love with it and am desperate to see it thrive and grow. So I put it in my sunniest window and diligently water it every day. And, each day as I water it, I think of how much I love this plant and its beautiful red flowers and revel in my affection for it. And yet, despite the love in my heart, after a week or two, this beautiful creature is right and truly dead. I am heartbroken and think terrible thoughts about myself and how I can never keep anything I love alive. Maybe I vow to never again accept such a beautiful plant into my care.

What actually happened? I watered my beautiful plant with my love and affection. Why wasn't that enough?

It wasn't enough because I never actually entered into a loving *relationship* with the plant. Instead, I poured my deluded certainty about what love should look like on it, but I never actually got to know this particular and unique living being.

So let's try this again. This time, when I receive the beautiful, flowering plant from my loved one, I look closely at its leaves and flowers and acknowledge that this precious being is a mystery to me. I acknowledge that I have a great deal to learn about how to skillfully care for it and that my affection, by itself, is not sufficient. So I set off, with loving intention, to learn as much as I can about how to nurture this particular plant. I hungrily search out knowledge on the internet. I talk to friends and neighbors. Maybe I learn that this particular plant only thrives in indirect sunlight and only wants to be watered once a week at most.

With these guidelines, I start to take more skillful care of my beloved plant, and, most importantly, to pay very close attention to what my plant is telling me on a day-to-day basis about how it is doing and what causes it to thrive or to suffer. I notice its leaves and how they're looking. I touch the soil to find out how it feels, if it is ready for more water or still soaking in nutrients. I invite it to teach me, and I bow to its teaching. This is the point at which I have entered into the *practice* of love.

Love Languages

You have probably heard that people have different love languages. Though there is some emerging evidence to support this idea in the scientific literature, the story of love languages is most compelling to us because it communicates what feels like an important and fundamental truth. It is one of the truths that we are pointing to here in this chapter—that sometimes how we ourselves receive love is not how our partner best receives love.

The author who originally coined the term *love languages,* Gary Chapman, posits that what makes each of us feel most loved can be different in somewhat predictable ways. For some people, *getting gifts* makes them feel seen, appreciated, and loved. For others, *words of affection* and admiration, such as "I love you" and "I think you're amazing" are what makes them feel most loved and well supported. For yet others, it is *physical touch* that helps them feel their partner's affection, attraction, care, and love. Other folks yearn for *acts of service*—things done that communicate "I see what you need help with, and I gladly lend my hand to lift your burden." Finally, for some others, love is *time*; for example, "I know you love me because you spend your time with me."

For me, the most important teaching in Chapman's work is that we tend to give love in the form that we most like to receive love. For example, if my love language is time together, I will show my partner love by spending lots of time with her. Similarly, if I were a fern, the kind that desires to be misted with water every day, I would care for my partner plant by misting her every day—even if she were a cactus. And there is the rub: When we approach loving our partner informed only by our own wants and needs, we inadvertently only reinforce our own ego and our own delusion of separateness.

In here is also a valuable lesson about humility. We are invited to consider the possibility, even the likelihood, that we don't actually have any idea what makes our partner feel most loved. Or that if we were lucky enough to know yesterday, we may no longer know today. We must carry the question like a *koan*. A koan is a kind of living question that we take up as a gateway into the great unfolding mystery of life. It is a question that we only ever provisionally know the answer to, a question that must be answered anew every day—in this case, our koan is "My darling, how do I best love you today?"

Here is where we begin the practice of cultivating our intention.

When we approach loving our partner informed only by our own wants and needs, we inadvertently only reinforce our own ego and our own delusion of separateness.

Setting the Intention to Love Skillfully

It is so easy in our relationships to let ourselves fall into operating on autopilot, mindlessly making our way through the day. We let our partner simply become another object in the field that we are only half paying attention to—if that. We react *to* them, rather than act *toward* them with awareness and care.

The antidote is learning to love skillfully, and that, as with all things, begins with intention: the intention to grow in our capacity to love our partner, to love ourselves, and to love all beings. Both the attitude and the practice are things that we can be wholly responsible for, because they are completely within us, and they do not depend on the worthiness of others. This is where we first take up the relational practice of loving-kindness, also known as *maitri.*

In the practice of loving-kindness, we gather ourselves into the moment, breathing deeply and feeling our way into awareness of the present moment, settling into our body, and opening ourselves to receive all the arisings of the moment—body, mind, and heart. We want to be fully present when we set our intention, so that we aren't just mouthing words mindlessly and without weight. In other words, we want to bring ourselves and our intention into focus so that we mean what we say when we say it.

Then we bring our partner to mind. If they are present, we look at them. If they aren't present, we might use a picture of them or simply invite their image into our mind. Then, using the words that follow, or others of our own, we cultivate our heartfelt desire for our partner to experience love and well-being:

May you, my dear, on this day feel healthy, radiant, and well.
May your mind be at ease—bright, sharp, and clear.
May you feel loved and treasured.
May your heart be at peace and feel full and content.
May you experience joy and be delighted by many things.
May your eyes light up and your heart gladden.
May you be happy and at ease.
May your gifts be a boundless treasure for all beings.

The intention is to consciously set our loving-kindness relationship goal for the day. In this intention-setting practice, we deliberately wipe the scales of habit from our eyes and set our determination to see our partner clearly, with fresh eyes, and to take up our commitment to their love and well-being with seriousness and vigor.

May you feel loved and treasured, happy, and at ease.

Spiritually, we want to practice in such a way that we begin to lower the barrier between self and other—to see for ourselves that the ego concern that separates us diminishes us both. We set the intention to realize our partner's happiness as our very own. We set the intention to do whatever we can to bring them joy and alleviate their suffering, because they are not separate from us, and their well-being is our own. If we genuinely feel our way into this, we already know this to be a fundamental truth. When our partner suffers, we suffer. When our partner is well, we are well. We are not-two, and this not-two arises, here and now, endlessly.

Paying Attention to How Our Partner Wants to Receive Love

Love as a spiritual practice arises out of the cultivation of compassionate understanding and sympathetic joy. Out of truly understanding your partner's ten thousand joys and sorrows. This part of the practice involves cultivating our capacity for sustained attention and deep looking. As with our plant analogy, when we were looking closely at the leaves to receive their teaching about what makes the plant thrive or suffer, we practice paying close attention to our partner to notice for ourselves what helps them to feel loved and well.

For example, this might be the practice by which we learn what our partner's actual love language is. Most directly, we could simply ask and take our partner at their word, but we might also pay attention and learn for ourself, because life is made of subtleties. What makes our partner's eyes light up? What makes them smile, or laugh with joy?

For folks for whom gifts are their love language, it might be that flowers and candy bring them joy, but even for them, it is often the thoughtfulness of the gift that really communicates love. I find that it helps to first set the intention that I want to give my partner a gift versus thinking that I have to buy a present. The latter is obligatory, but the first is genuinely loving and generous. Then we simply pay attention to what our partner says and does over the course of a small handful of days. We will often find that the answer arrives effortlessly, as our partner shows us what they want or need or dream of. Maybe it's something they say about wanting a new book to read, or missing their horses, or how delighted they are when their dogs play with their toys. Gifts abound. You simply need to pay attention.

But, of course, this is best applied to partners who genuinely receive gifts as acts of love. Some people are really not moved by gifts at all. And yet we might give them anyway, because that is our habit, or the habit imposed on us by our culture. This speaks to the practice of careful attention. Living with intention, if you discover that someone you love does not receive love through gifts, you might make your gift in the form of their actual love language. Perhaps an act of service or simply time together.

For example, my mother, in her 90s at the time of this writing, doesn't really need or want for much these days. Honestly, upon reflection, she's never really been the sort of person who lights up when she receives gifts. Yet for years I have given her gifts every year for all of the noteworthy holidays like Mother's Day, Christmas, and her birthday. And, inevitably, she always tells me, well in advance, "Jim, don't worry about getting me anything. I already have more than I need." She is invariably gracious when I do give her something, but it has become more and more clear that this just isn't her love language. What is her love language? Well, as it turns out, it's acts of service. At her age, legally blind, and quite hard of hearing, she can't really take care of all the things she used to do. I've taken over many tasks for her, such as paying her bills, filing her taxes, making meals, getting groceries, sending cards, and housecleaning. And this is what I've noticed: For these small acts of service, my mother lights up and says, "Thank you" in the most genuine and heartfelt way, and it is so clear that she feels loved and cared for. Now I know. And I am so grateful. So grateful to finally know how best to love this woman who has loved me so unconditionally for my whole life. Blessings abound.

Our partners, our friends, our parents, all the people that we love in the world, do not come with instruction manuals, and so we must set out to discover them for ourselves. If you had to write the manual for your partner about what makes them tick, could you do it? As you begin to engage this practice of careful and loving attention, I guarantee you will be better and better able to do so.

The Single Hand

The key to this kind of attention as a spiritual practice is cultivating it as an utterly selfless act; allowing, if just for the moment, that our partner's suffering is the only suffering that matters. Our partner's happiness is the only happiness that matters. To let our own ego fall away. To no longer see our partner as other, but as not separate. In this practice of attention, we cultivate not-separate, not as an idea or a romantic notion, but as a genuinely felt sense—palpable, embodied, obvious, and undeniable.

Thich Nhat Hanh notes that, just as the right hand immediately comes to the aid of the left hand when it is injured with no thought of being separate, we are moved to care for our partner just as naturally and just as effortlessly. When we let our attention dissolve us into wholeness, then we realize that it is only ever the right hand that tends the left, and the left hand that tends the right. There is only ever tending and being tended. There is only ever this single hand.

BEING THE LEFT HAND

Paying mindful attention is an essential component of cultivating loving-kindness as a practice. Aim to do so as a selfless, loving act.

1. When you and your partner are together, commit to spending 15 minutes paying attention only to your partner's experience.
2. Take a deep breath and let it out slowly as you let go of your own perspective and imagine your way into your partner's mind and body. What are they experiencing right now? What do you imagine they are feeling? Happy? Sad? Stressed? Upset? Content? What do you imagine they are feeling in their body? Tense? Relaxed? Warm? Cold? What do you imagine they are thinking about?
3. Now, knowing that they are the right hand and you are the left, how will you move to be of aid, comfort, and support? Do they need you to say something loving and encouraging? Would they enjoy a cup of tea or a cold drink? Do they need help with a problem or chore? In this moment, your partner is the only person that matters in the whole world. The purpose of your entire existence is their well-being. Just for these few minutes, give yourself completely to that goal.
4. Let your ego dissolve in the service of selfless attention. Notice where there is resistance arising in you, and simply allow that resistance to flow through you without grasping onto it. Stay tuned in to your partner and release yourself into their service.
5. Breathe.

Our Cups Are Not Separate

When we are experiencing our relationship from a place of separateness, rather than a place of wholeness, we think that we are taking something away from ourselves when we give, sacrificing *our* resources, being diminished, even if it is coming from a place of generosity. From this place of separateness, we are being generous with our resources—but we experience them as *our* resources, which we could have spent on ourselves. So we have taken something away from ourselves to give it to our partner, whether that be time, energy, money, or any other seemingly limited resource. From our normal, if deluded, perspective of separation, generosity is taking out of one cup to fill another.

When we are practicing paying attention to learn how to best and most effectively love our partner (or any other being), our attention must instead be rooted not in generosity but in true intimacy, connection, and interwovenness. The idea is that we are not pouring from our cup into our partner's; we are simply filling this cup from the bounty of the universe.

We are never taking anything away; we are only adding. As Rumi notes, we are not drops in the ocean; we are the ocean itself. We do not have individual and separate cups that require guarding and constant attention and "self-care" to fill up; rather, we are interwoven from the same context, poured together into the same cup, woven from the same cloth, comprised of the same stars, born from the same universe.

So this place from which giver, receiver, and gift are just this one thing, this is the place to which we root our attention when we set out to discover how to love our partner with skill and wisdom. We do this for the love of our partner. We do this for our own awakening and liberation. We do this in service to all beings. We want to grow beyond the simple intent to nurture optimal relationship health. In the realm of awakening to true intimacy, in the realm of the spirit, this genuinely selfless love is the love at the heart of the universe, waiting to free us.

We are not pouring from our cup into our partner's; we are simply filling this cup from the bounty of the universe.

So we pay attention, and while we are paying attention, we notice any resistance that arises. This resistance is, more than likely, the ego arising to assert its place in the field of separateness. The bite of the separate self. The hook that keeps us trapped in suffering. It is the selfish imp of "what about me?" And, if we pay really close attention, we might start to recognize for ourself just how often the "what about me?" impulse is lawfully followed by intense suffering for both ourselves and our partner. In my experience, "what about me?" very rarely leads to wise and compassionate action. Which is not to say that our own health, safety, and well-being are not equally deserving of our care and compassion. It's just that, more often than not, it is the fear and vulnerability that keep us so heavily invested in our own separateness.

Attention is the most basic form of love. In the service of loving-kindness, practicing mindful attention means paying good, close, loving attention to what makes our partner thrive. The next step is enacting what we've learned with intention and skill.

In the service of loving-kindness, practicing mindful attention means paying good, close, loving attention to what makes our partner thrive.

Skillful Action: Communicating in the Language of Love

Once we have set our intention to realize that our partner is not separate from us and have taken up the practice of paying close and loving attention to their joys and sorrows (as not separate from our own), we begin to put what we are learning into practice. From within deepening understanding and insight, we begin to create the mystery of love with skill and grace. Rather than inadvertently falling into a pattern in which our partner feels neglected, trapped, or controlled, we skillfully cultivate the actions that allow our partner to feel supported, free, loved, joyful, strong, capable, competent, and a source of healing in the world.

As discussed in previous chapters, enacting the practice of serving the well-being of our partner involves the embodied experience of learning by doing. We move in the world, and the world responds. We then learn from and are shaped by that response. We are in and of the world and are constantly changing and being changed by it. We are in and of the unfolding of relationship with our partner, and we are constantly changing and being changed by them. This is intimacy.

So from that place of interdependent co-arising, from the place where we are actively co-creating each other, we do our best to move in ways that alleviate our partner's suffering and enhance their joy, happiness, and well-being. Then we notice the results of our efforts and adjust as necessary.

RECEIVING AND RESPONDING TO LOVING-KINDNESS

Love as a practice involves a lot of trial-and-error learning. Encourage yourself to just try something and then simply notice how it is received.

- **Let your partner's well-being be your teacher**. Allow yourself to be shaped by those teachings. Begin by simply noticing. Ask yourself, How can I water the seeds of my partner's happiness and joy? What makes their eyes light up? What makes them feel loved, secure, joyful, peaceful, and content? How might I be an agent of intimacy, nurturance, and safety in their life?
- **Notice your partner's reception.** Time together, acts of service, gifts, physical affection, words of affirmation—try them all at different times, in different contexts, during different moods or phases of the moon. As you try each (I offer dozens of ideas in the "Heart of the Matter" at the end of this chapter), notice the response you get from your partner. Are they happy or delighted? Grateful? Are they, instead, perhaps only politely grateful, but not particularly pleased? Or maybe your offering is unnoticed or even unwelcome. Any of these outcomes is a sacred response.
- **Pay close attention.** Just noticing and making a note of their response is how we begin. This is where journaling can be handy. Write down what you've noticed today about the things that make your partner's eyes light up, the things that soothe their aching heart, that bring them comfort and ease their mind. This ongoing exploration should be fun and should feel generous and loving. This is how we learn to love what matters.
- **Notice your response**. In turn, you might choose to practice with and learn from your own reactions. Noticing how you might be delighted when your gift brings your partner joy. Noticing how you might be disappointed, hurt, defensive, or even angry if your gift is not well received. How do you, who have taken up the practice of awakening, receive and respond to these arisings?

All of this doing will lead to, perhaps, awareness of your shared joy. You can then notice that the seeds of your generosity are watered, and you become an even more enthusiastic servant to the well-being of others. Perhaps you more deeply realize that there are no others, but only this.

We might also notice the constriction that arises when our offering is not well received. This may be the hook of our ego, taking it personally, rising up in umbrage to either fight or flee. In this moment, we might meet our constriction with love and attention, caring for it gently and loosening the knots we tie ourselves in so that we might reconnect with our generous and interconnected heart. To love skillfully, we must learn to host our anger and hurt, our fight or flight, skillfully so that we might refrain from harm. We might then notice that this offering, in this moment, simply does not serve. Moving forward, we enact our vow to continue learning by doing.

The Heart of the Matter

We offer our time. We offer our presence. We offer our ear. We offer our service. We offer our gifts. We offer our vulnerability. We offer our truth and our hearts. We offer our loving touch. We offer our passion. We offer our sexuality. We offer our sensuality. We offer the shirt off our back. We offer our need. We offer our heartache. We offer the stars, and the grass, and the wind in the trees. We offer brown, and birdsong, and the smoke from spent candles. We offer shoelaces and barking dogs and the space between breaths. We offer everything. We offer everything.

We offer everything.

This is what we do in the name of skillful loving action. We wash the dishes. We walk the dogs. We dry the tears. We comfort the heartache. We talk about the future. We make plans. We express gratitude. We jump bones. We make love. We share memories. We make more. We clean up messes. We mow the grass. We share popcorn from the same bowl. We make breakfast. We serve coffee. We catch spiders (and move them outside). We hold hands. We sit in the waiting room. We kiss the scars. We admire their beauty and their brilliance. We stop to smell the lilacs. We rub the feet. We pass the tissues. We search for the lost phone. We talk about everything, and nothing. We say, "I love you!" over and over, every day, all day, in all the ways we know how, spoken and unspoken, 108 times a day.

And we learn how to love, with skill and presence. Always and forever. Amen.

Mindful Mantra

May you be well.
May you be happy.
May you feel loved and treasured.
May you know peace.
May you be a light in the darkness for others.
And may I be a source of joy and comfort to you for all the days of my life.

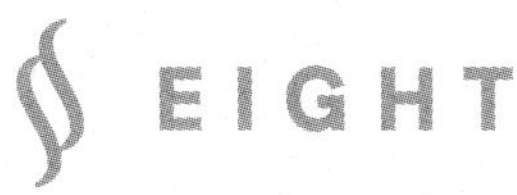

EIGHT

The Red Thread

SEX AND THE PATH OF PHYSICAL INTIMACY

Why can't even the most enlightened person sever the red thread of passion?
—As quoted by Judith Ragir of the Clouds in Water Zen Center

If we want to practice the path of true intimacy, that path must include becoming unabashedly intimate with our shared sexual nature, with such brilliant clarity and love that all shame and shadow are illuminated and the barriers between ourselves and our partner dissolve into a vibrant wholeness. In this chapter, we refer to "sexual nature" as the "red thread of passion." Through our contemplative practice, we can become intimate with the red thread in ways that not only do no harm but also serve both the health of our relationships and the awakening of our own true nature.

The Problem of Separateness

Unhappiness with their sexual relationship is frequently among the most significant concerns that couples report to both relationship scientists and therapists. Considered through the lens of our intimacy practice, it is within the domain of our sexual relationship that we tend to feel most exquisitely vulnerable. Vulnerable to rejection. Vulnerable to judgment—both our partner's and perhaps especially our own. Vulnerable to feelings of shame, embarrassment, and failure. And as is our experience with all our vulnerabilities, our instinct is to turn away from and escape our vulnerable feelings as quickly and thoroughly as possible, whether that escape takes the form of fight or flight.

Our experience of our sexuality is so fraught with vulnerability, and often trauma, that we commonly find ways to distance ourselves from that incredible tenderness. We all find our own secret ways to both approach sex and, simultaneously, avoid intimacy. To be physically present, but mentally, emotionally, and spiritually distant. We each, over the course of our lives and experiences, acquire our own repertoires of separation, so that we might find some way to engage our sexual natures without exposing our true, whole, authentic, and vulnerable selves.

I would argue that all suffering within sexual relationships arises from turning away from vulnerability and intimacy. Relationship scientists know from decades of research that up to a quarter of all couples are unhappy with their sexual relationship. According to a large 2017 survey study in the *Archives of Sexual Behavior* by Jean H. Kim, Wilson S. Tam, and Peter Muennig, approximately 20% of couples in the United States report being in a sexless relationship—defined as a relationship in which the couple has sex less than 10 times per year. Researchers also have discovered that partners generally only know about half of the things their partner likes sexually and only about a quarter of what they definitely don't like. Turning away from vulnerability leads to us knowing too little about ourselves and each other sexually, which then leads us to turning away from sex altogether, which then leaves us separate, alone, and unhappy.

When we consider the factors that appear to negatively affect couples' satisfaction with their sexual relationship, we notice that all of these factors involve turning away from each other and ourselves. For example, many couples experience some form of diagnosable sexual dysfunction, including difficulties with arousal, pain, desire, and orgasm. However, these physical issues appear to corrode emotional and sexual intimacy only when they lead to a constriction of couples' sensual and sexual engagement. And, perhaps more

Turning away from vulnerability leads to us knowing too little about ourselves and each other sexually, which then leads us to turning away from sex altogether, which then leaves us separate, alone, and unhappy.

important, when they exacerbate couples' reluctance to talk openly, kindly, and collaboratively about their sexual relationship.

Additionally, there is growing evidence that pornography use has a corrosive effect on sexual and relationship satisfaction for both partners, not only because it is a readily available avenue for turning away from the relationship but also because pornography creates an insulated mental and emotional container within which sexual desire is imprisoned away from an authentic and vibrant sexual relationship with another real and vividly engaged human being.

When we consider also what we know about the factors that appear to positively affect couples' sexual satisfaction, we notice that all these factors involve turning toward each other to care for the relationship and to be open, vulnerable, and authentic about ourselves as sexual beings. These nurturing factors of sexual intimacy include couples' overall relationship satisfaction, the quality of their sexual communication, the degree to which they talk about what they like and don't like, the degree to which they create feelings of emotional connection before, during, and after sex, the degree to which both partners feel safe and invited to initiate sex, and the degree to which partners are generously attentive to each other's pleasure.

Pornography and the I–It Relationship

As we consider our lived experience of sexuality and the habits that can undermine intimacy through turning away, one important step is to divest ourselves of the images and stories that reinforce a dualistic view of self and other in the expression of our sexuality. In his 1971 book, *I and Thou*, the philosopher Martin Buber draws our attention to the variety of ways in which we relate to others in relationship. He draws a distinction for us between ways of relating in which we regard the other as an object or a thing (an I–It relationship) and ways of relating in which we regard the other as fully human but perhaps still separate (an I–You relationship), and, finally, ways of relating in which we regard the other as sacred (an I–Thou relationship). In the I–Thou relationship the other is not a separate object to which one relates; instead, there is only the emergent relationship—"I" does not exist independent of "Thou."

With this series of distinctions, Buber leads us through considering that the attitude that we bring to our most important relationships can span the gamut from dangerously objectifying through commonly dualistic and thus normatively othering to an honoring of the sacred and mysterious. Within our intimacy practice, we might go even a step further in drawing our attention to the possibility of seeing through the remaining duality of I–Thou to the wholly nonseparated experience of true nondual union, in which there is no self and no other, but instead the holistic experience of only just this vividly unfolding moment.

So if the intention of our spiritual practice is to diminish the pernicious barriers that lead us to feel separate from others, it may benefit our practice to consider asking what those domains of experience are that reinforce the walls of separation and destructive othering. Though there are many places where we learn to objectify and "other" the people in our lives, in the realm of sexuality one of the primary culprits in our culture is pornography. We might also include the effects on our minds of some movies, TV shows, articles, and "locker room talk" that dehumanize people as sexual objects. We are drawn to these narratives of separation because they are pervasive, because they are, by their nature, sexually enticing, and because, honestly, we simply are not attentive to the potential spiritual damage that they can do.

These "I–It" ways of being can be uniquely harmful forms of self-protection. We can use them as ways of suppressing and removing the vulnerability inherent in sexuality and instead covering that vulnerability with dominance, harshness, anger, bitterness, and objectification.

I do not mean to create feelings of shame or judgment. We are products of our histories and circumstances, and we arrive where we arrive for understandable reasons. However, I do want to invite us to simply consider the consequences of porn for the path of spiritual awakening within our sexually intimate relationships. So much pornography sullies the beauty and worth of the people involved. More importantly, porn by its very nature is nonrelational and thus can only ever cultivate an I–It mind set. And cultivation of a cognitive habit for experiencing our sexuality within an I–It frame diminishes our capacity to fully arrive inside of, and dissolve ourselves within, an unfolding sexual moment.

For example, habitual consumption of sexual imagery, whether through video or text, creates images, fantasies, and expectations within the mind that are then available as a basis for comparison during actual moments of relational sexuality. In turn, it splits our attention between the actual moment and the imagined moment and diminishes our availability to our partner and our actual lived experience within the unfolding moment. In other words, when we are having sex with our partner, most of our attention may be on the images and fantasies in our head and thus unavailable for the vividness and brilliance that is a moment of sexual union.

There is a well-known phenomenon in the clinical treatment of sexual dysfunction known as *spectatoring*. Spectatoring, as a phenomenon, is characterized by getting stuck in a third-person perspective when having sex. The person cannot fully enter the moment because in essence they are watching themselves have sex instead of losing themselves in the physicality and sensuality of the sexual act. Some of the predictable consequences of spectatoring are diminished enjoyment, erectile dysfunction, shame, disappointment, and dissatisfaction for both partners. This can be a difficult experience to address. However, apropos of the point I am hoping to make here, successful treatment involves practices that help the person draw their attention back into the moment-to-moment unfolding of their actual lived experience without judgment, comparison, or spectatoring. As it turns out, this is easier said than done and can require a great deal of practice and patience as the person slowly replaces an overpracticed mental habit with a newer and healthier practice of presence.

Turning Away from Our Sexual Selves

Resolving the dilemma of wanting to express our sexual selves without experiencing our vulnerability often leads us to suppress or deny our sexual feelings. Suppression and denial of our sexual selves can be dangerous in at least a couple of ways. First, we cannot integrate and work skillfully with anything we are suppressing. A great deal of sexual misconduct arises from just this lack of integration. Second, suppression and denial are often accompanied by shame and guilt, cutting us off from a fundamental aspect of our common humanity. A spiritual practice cannot be truly fruitful if any part of who we are is not attended to fully and considered deeply. Thus our progress along the intimate path requires that we attend with love, care, and diligence to the full range of our own sexual experience, for the care of ourselves and all beings. It is exactly through this diligent and compassionate attention that we are able to cultivate the most skillful and beneficent action in the field of the red thread.

Traditional manifestations of Buddhism and other spiritual traditions have found themselves cordoning off sex and sexuality from spiritual practice for many reasons, only one of which is the incredible power that our sexual appetites have to elicit both greed and aversion, which in turn fairly inevitably leads to inner turmoil and external harm causing.

For example, greed arises in the form of lust, which, when left to its own devices and allowed to steer the ship, can result in great harm to ourselves and others. From a place of undigested greed, we become willing to harm, devalue, exploit, manipulate, or use others to satiate the urgency of our yearning. Rather than being able to experience sexual yearning intimately—with awareness, joy, and compassion as simply another vivid human arising in the moment—we turn away from it by seeking only its immediate gratification. It is from this place that people so often abuse their power to feed their own sexual appetites. In relationship, greed most easily manifests as selfishness, in which we want sex for ourselves with an exclusive focus on our own release and little regard for our partner's experience of arousal or pleasure. We feel entitled to what we want when we want it and feel resentful when we don't get it. Greed, because it is self-focused, leads to treating our partner as an object for the satisfaction of our yearning rather than as our beloved other whose experience of pleasure and love matter deeply to us.

Our progress along the intimate path requires that we attend with love, care, and diligence to the full range of our own sexual experience.

Similarly, aversion arises in the form of fear and resentment of rejection, which we are hardwired to experience as incredibly painful and easily perceive as "unacceptable." From a place of undigested aversion, we can lash out in anger, rage, self-pity, and heartlessness to avenge our sense of hurt and injustice. We turn away from our vulnerability by armoring it with anger and resentment, or by denying, suppressing, or withdrawing from the vivid experiencing of our sexual longing. It is from this place that some people then act out their resentment and anger through violence, belittling, degrading, or exploiting others, toxically mixing their sexuality with contempt and rage. In relationship, aversion to our own sexuality or to our vulnerability to rejection can manifest as both anger and withdrawal. We might treat our partner's sexuality or sexual independence with contempt or simply withdraw and avoid our sexual relationship altogether.

Sexuality becomes something of the "third rail" in our spiritual psychology, because its power is so ancient and vast that it can appear virtually uncontrollable, thus requiring a lot of external boundaries, rules, and vigilance. This dedicated external control is clearly advisable and necessary in the day-to-day lives we live in community with each other. However, in the context of our spiritual lives, whatever we avoid and cordon off only serves to further split us off from the divine. In the practice of a path that takes up intimacy as both the means and the end of the spiritual life, we must integrate our sexual nature as an inseparable facet of our inherent worthiness, our true nature, and our inherent wholeness. Through our mindfulness practice, as we learn to encounter our naturally occurring sexual feelings and fear of rejection with compassionate attention and spaciousness, we can then experience the arising of sexual feelings without denial while still behaving in skillful ways that do the most good and the least harm.

Reclaiming Our Sexuality

> Nicco and Yumi have fallen out of the habit of expressing physical affection and intimacy within their relationship. Both of them have noticed this lack of connection in their lives, and Yumi in particular has started to worry that she isn't being perceived as attractive anymore. On a rare opportunity for a date night, Yumi chooses to wear a particularly sexy top. You know, the kind that is well made, flattering, and just the right amount of revealing. She feels confident and hopeful about rekindling a spark in their relationship. They go out to their favorite restaurant and have a nice dinner. They spend the entire night talking and enjoying one another's company. And yet, Nicco never comments on how Yumi looks. They get home, and Nicco immediately changes into comfortable clothes and turns on the TV. Working up her courage, Yumi gives it another try, snuggling up against Nicco so their shoulders are touching and fingers intertwined. Nicco gives Yumi's hand a sweet little squeeze and turns up the volume on the TV.

This example shows us how easy it can be for us to get caught up in the habits of daily living, to the detriment of the vividly lived experience of the moment. We don't really know where Nicco's attention is, but we can guess it is caught up in the many details of their lives, none of which are present currently in these precious few moments with Yumi. Whatever sensuality may be vividly apparent is veiled behind the habits we acquire to pay attention almost solely to the irritants of the past and future. Yumi, for her part, is also not wholly present to the vividness of the unfolding moment. Though to some degree she is with Nicco, she is also actively carrying an expectation of how she wants the evening to go and how she wants Nicco to be and is distracted from the actual moment by repeatedly comparing what is actually happening to her expectation of what *should* be happening. In many ways, these are the basic ingredients for our very human experience of disappointment. The opportunity for vibrancy is lost to the degree that we are not wholly present.

Breathing Life Into Our Sexual Relationship

Our sexual relationship is available to us as a gateway into the universal truth, into presence, into awakening from the delusion of separation—if we are willing to enter it as such. If we are willing to enter it with our whole being.

The domain of sex, sexuality, sensuality, lust, and passion is challenging for most of us in our practice—both intrapersonal and interpersonal. How each of us comes to relate to our experience of the red thread—sexual passion on the intimate path—is an inescapable facet of the path of wisdom and compassion. In turn, how we learn to enact our sexual passion in relationship is an essential component of a truly intimate and interwoven connection.

I suspect that the bizarre double-bind messages about sex and sexuality that most of us heard growing up—in a culture that represses our sexual nature and then endlessly stimulates that nature to sell us things—trapped us between enforced ignorance and the image of wanton engagement as a commodity. In turn, it drove many to greet the powerful waves of sexual energy that are part of being human with shame and secrecy. Not knowing what to do with the red thread, many of us can have great difficulty reconciling our sexuality with all the other aspects of our lives into a sense of wholeness, integrity, confidence, and peace.

When the red thread of passion is left in the dark—uneducated, unexamined, and repeatedly hooked into the wild west of what can be sold and leveraged—then it can, and too often does, emerge to be enacted in harmful ways. We become ghosts of separation, turning away, lost in a world of self and other. We become lost in a world in which others are simply objects in the unfolding of our sexual confusion. We are lost, lonely, and perpetually unsatisfied, and we collude in such a way that everyone else we encounter is lost, lonely, and perpetually unsatisfied.

And yet, the domain of the red thread is rightly and truly a gateway to wholeness, intimacy, integrity, passion, and joy.

Setting the Intention to Turn toward the Red Thread

In Rumi's poem *Like This,* he shows how our sexuality is inseparable from a life of wholeness in the moment. In the poem he writes that, if someone asks us what the perfect satisfaction of all our sexual wanting looks like, we simply lift our face and say *like this.*

Union. Wholeness. Intimacy. Just this.

This is the domain of both spirit and soul—that which reaches up to become one with the brightness and that which reaches down into the earth, becoming one with the dark. It is the goal of our contemplative practice to uncover and unleash it. To melt away the barriers that separate us. To meet here, in the field of intimacy.

So how do we take up this practice of wholeness? How do we find our way to the integration of our sensual and sexual nature into the rich fabric of our lives?

First, let's begin with a moment of orientation—by considering our intention. And here in the realm of the red thread, the intention is presence. We might start with the intention: *I want to be fully and attentively present.* The intention is union. *I want to see through the barrier of self and other into the vibrancy of us and thus.* The intention is awakening. Awakening from the illusion of separateness to the vividness of true intimacy.

So, as we set out on *this* path, as we engage relationship as a genuinely spiritual practice, we first gently set the intention to turn toward wholeness, to turn toward authenticity, to turn toward the vulnerability of full presence, to enter the moment with trust and faith—in ourselves and in each other. Of course, the enactment and actualization of full presence is easier said than done, and that is why it must be engaged as an ongoing *practice.*

Because it is so common in our culture to think of sex in terms of goals we imagine we *should* achieve, such as erection, lubrication, and orgasm, the intention to turn toward must also include turning toward what is *actually* unfolding in this moment of sexuality with our partner. In this practice, we will want to, perhaps gradually, begin to diminish our allegiance to our expectations and our compulsions to achieve. In fact, bringing the mind of achievement into the realm of sexual intimacy is radically counterproductive.

Instead, the intention is simply to practice presence. To practice with love, gentleness, compassion, and patience. We will find the edge of our vulnerability, over and over again, and the work is to simply feel our way into that edge with loving and patient attention. The edge I mean here is the point at which our experience of present-hearted vulnerability begins to overwhelm us and we begin to withdraw from the intensity of our sexual experience or fear of rejection to some safer emotional distance.

Our edge may be our hesitation to talk about sex with our partner or our reluctance to initiate or communicate what we want or don't want. Or our edge might be a fear of letting go fully into the vibrancy of our sexual experience. Or our edge might be turning toward the experience of embarrassment that arises when we believe we've failed in some way sexually so that we might connect and recover the ongoing moment of sensuality.

The key to caring for our edge is nonhostility. We must not attack our edge, nor condemn or judge it. We must simply know it and hold it, acknowledge and host it, and invite it to soften, or even just consider softening, if only for a breath or a heartbeat. We approach the practice of presence knowing that it may be slow going, that it will involve stepping forward (even tentatively) and then stepping back, and that gentleness and self-compassion are key.

MEETING OUR EDGE WITH PRESENCE

With faith and determination, we can return, again and again, to our intention. As vulnerable as it makes us feel, we can make the following vows:

- I vow to turn toward the experience of my own sexual longing when that is what is present—whether what is skillful in the moment is acting on that longing or simply allowing it to be present.

- I vow to turn toward my partner's experience of sexual longing when that is what is present—whether what is skillful in that moment is acting on that longing or simply honoring that longing without acting on it.
- I vow to turn toward open, honest, and clear communication about sex in my relationship so that I might dispel my ignorance and know more clearly my partner's (and my own) sexual likes and dislikes.
- I vow to turn toward my fear of rejection so that I might hold that experience with love and compassion while learning to behave with skill and wisdom.
- I vow to turn toward, with generosity and clear attention, my partner's experience of pleasure and arousal.
- I vow to turn toward my own vivid experience of pleasure and arousal.
- I vow to turn toward cultivating a vibrant field of sexuality that emerges from the shared and sacred space within which there is no separation between myself and my beloved, but only *just this*.
- Into the fabric of my life, I will weave the vibrancy of the red thread into the wholeness of being, for myself and all others, throughout space and time.

Paying Attention to the Red Thread

But what exactly should we be doing with our attention if our intention is cultivating our sexual relationship as a spiritual practice? We begin by gently and lovingly attending to everything that arises in our body, heart, and mind when any hint of sexuality is part of our experience of the moment. Ultimately, we want body, heart, and mind, together, to be fully present, clear, and undivided from the full experience of the moment. Of course, in practice, that is a lot to pay attention to. So, given that, it may be helpful to break it down just a bit.

We need to pay attention to what we are paying attention to. Sexual relationship as a spiritual practice requires that we notice when our attention is on other things, including our *ideas* about how things should be going, so that we can gently bring our attention back to what is real and true and vivid, right here, right now. Intimacy is available only in the moment.

Mary Oliver notes in her poem, "Wild Geese," that you only have to let the soft animal of your body love what it loves. On the path of sexual relationship as spiritual practice, we want to engage in the practice of fully arriving and being completely present. Part of that is being attentive to what is arising in our mind. When we notice what is arising in the mind, we can, perhaps, if we are lucky, gently bring our attention back to being fully present in our *body*. Just as in the breath meditation practice, when we notice that our attention has wandered away from our physical experience, we simply guide our attention back to the soft animal of our body, allowing it to love what it loves.

AWAKENING TO SENSUALITY

In the practice of being wholly attentive to the physical realm, having set your intention to arrive fully, guide your attention to the sensations and perceptions of your body in your body. Attune to the endless sensual arising in the constantly flowing moment. This is an act of radical acceptance, as you generously allow yourself to feel exactly how you are feeling without judgment or interference.

1. Ground your attention in the body, the experience of skin-to-skin contact, notice what you are feeling with all the delicate little nerve endings within every millimeter of your skin.
2. Ground your attention on what you are seeing in the moment. Bring your attention to your eyes and how the light plays off your partner's skin, how the curve and texture radiate into being.
3. Ground your attention on what you are hearing in the moment. The sound of breath and pleasure.
4. Ground your attention on what you are tasting and smelling in the moment. The incense of intimacy.
5. Enter the practice of mindful sexual intimacy, with all your senses, your skin cells, and nerve endings open, and be overwhelmed until there is only this flow of sensual experience released from any thought of self or other.
6. Drop away self-concern, drop away the imagination of your partner as separate, and allow yourself to dissolve into the oceanic experience of sexual intimacy.
7. Allow sensations to move into the foreground of awareness, inviting the self to drop away, until there is only just this intimate intensity. As each sensation arises, it is experienced fully. And, as each sensation passes

away, it is released thoroughly, creating room for the arising of the next moment of experiencing. And then the next. And then the next.

To awaken is to become the flow, and moments of sexual connection can be extraordinarily powerful.

Yumi, disappointed, stands up from the couch and starts to head toward the bedroom. In a moment of clarity, Nicco feels her absence, notices a slight twinge of the heart, looks up at Yumi, and is struck by how stunning she looks in that top. Nicco turns off the TV, follows Yumi into the bedroom, and gently draws her into an embrace. Nicco kisses her forehead and whispers, "You look especially breathtaking tonight." Yumi somewhat bashfully replies, "I thought you didn't notice." Nicco returns, "I definitely noticed. . . . I just didn't want to risk seeming disrespectful." Yumi whispers, "Appreciating my body isn't disrespectful. Why do you think I wore the top?" Nicco smiles and kisses Yumi more deeply. "If I wasn't paying close enough attention before, I am now," he says.

Skillful Action: Securing the Red Thread between You and Your Partner

Begin with Stillness

Skillful action begins with stillness. Deeply rooted in our practice of upright sitting, we continuously cultivate our capacity to meet the intensity of our red-thread moments with clarity, spaciousness, and stillness. Our sexual natures are woven through our being, desire and aversion arise endlessly, and we practice meeting each moment of that arising without turning away, with presence and clarity, and with the spaciousness to accept the presence of the red thread with neither the compulsion to grasp out of greed nor the compulsion to reject out of shame. As sexual energy arrives onboard, we practice recognizing it and remaining still, breathing in its presence, and remaining still, savoring the shared humanity of it, and remaining still. And then, from this place of stillness, we choose wisely, honoring our vows to create the most good and the least harm possible.

Early on in our relationship, I asked my partner if she wanted to join me on a meditation retreat by saying, "Want to be still and silent with me for a few days?" She replied, "With you? I'd rather be able to move. . . . and not be quiet." I appreciated this suggestively flirty reminder that, while stillness and silence have their place in our practice, so too do movement and sound, a full vibrant orchestra of connection and love.

When held in the container of a respectful and consenting relationship, we can leap through the red-thread gate into the full expression of our shared sexual nature—body, mind, and heart—into the vibrant flow of true intimacy. We, who choose to tread the path of true intimacy as the embodiment of the spiritual life, are called to embrace the totality of our human experience, including, and perhaps especially, the vibrancy and intensity of our sexuality.

Once we vow to do the most good and the least harm, then we must commit to fully embracing the vulnerability and intensity that characterize the experience of our sexuality. Finally, if we choose to enact our sexuality in relationship, it requires nurturing relationships that encourage, support, and promote the healthy integration of sexuality and sexual expression as a practice of intimacy, joy, and connection. Ideally, we nurture a relationship field within which we and our partner feel safe embodying our authentic and vulnerable sexual selves—a relationship of mutual respect, care, tenderness, nonjudgment, kindness, love, and joy.

What Happens Outside the Bedroom Happens Inside the Bedroom

As it turns out, relationship satisfaction and sexual satisfaction are deeply intertwined. If we want to have a vibrant sex life, we have to take good and loving care of all the other moments in our relationship. Similarly, if we want to have a happy relationship, we have to take good and loving care of sexual connection. The chemistry of sexual connection is always, always being affected by everything we do and say throughout the day.

They say that sexual connection at night begins with emotional connection in the morning. In fact, sexual connection in our intimate relationship began when we first laid eyes on each other and continues to be affected by every word and deed, all day, every day. Many of us make the mistake of believing that our sexual relationship is separate from the rest of our relationship, somehow siloed off and unaffected by all the other aspects of our relationship. But our lived experience tells us, if we are willing to listen to it, that what happens outside of the bedroom cannot be separated from what happens inside the bedroom. Not only does this mean that if you are harsh and shabby to each other throughout the day, it is going to have a harsh and shabby effect on your sex life, but equally that if we are dismissive and neglectful of our sexual connection, it is going to have an inescapably corrosive effect on our intimate connection throughout the rest of our relationship. This is simply the lived truth of cause and effect and interdependent co-arising.

Therefore, engage your mindfulness practice with consistency and determination to nurture the ground within which you deeply root a healthy and satisfying relationship. Study closely all the chapters of this book and joyfully engage the practice of intimacy—loving attention, deep listening, healthy attachment. Everything you do all day, every day, to strengthen your intimate connection will strengthen your sexual connection as well.

Skillful Communication

According to a 2020 review by Allen Mallory in the *Journal of Family Psychology*, one of the most consistent findings in the research and clinical literature is that the couples who communicate the most easily and clearly about sex—before, during, and after—have the most satisfying sex lives. However, we also know that the vast majority of couples have a really hard time talking about sex with each other. The taboo, shame, and embarrassment engendered by our culture are so powerful that, for the most part, partners remain silent to the point of being functionally mute. Interestingly, according to a 2017 review of the literature by Sharon Scales Rostosky and Ellen D. B. Riggle in *Psychology of Sexual Orientation and Gender Diversity*, research also finds that this is most commonly an issue for heterosexual couples and that same-sex couples are significantly more communicative about sex (and thus generally measurably more satisfied with their sex lives).

In our practice of nurturing ever deeper intimacy with ourselves and each other, the practice of open and clear communication about sex is a very powerful intimacy practice.

It requires us to openheartedly encounter and gently hold the enormous vulnerability that arises for us and our partner, meeting hesitation and reluctance with compassion and gentle encouragement. It calls on us to hold our own powerful emotions of fear of rejection, embarrassment, and shame with great care, while simultaneously encouraging ourselves to take the risk of saying out loud what we have so carefully kept to ourselves, to turn toward and explore what we have so assiduously avoided. It also requires us to meet with openhearted acceptance whatever our partner shares with us. If we want to nurture a space in our sexual relationship in which we both feel safe, comfortable, and generously invited to communicate openly, then we have to meet even the most tentative or awkward attempts with love and joy.

Open communication means that you will also discover the whole range of your likes, dislikes, and curiosities. Some of those you will have in common and some you will not. Like co-creating a Venn diagram of two separate but overlapping circles, you and your partner are collaborating toward a clear understanding of where your circles overlap, as well as a clear understanding of where they don't. Where they overlap—joy. Where they do not—generosity, collaboration, and honest boundaries.

Given that open sexual communication is incredibly difficult for most couples, this has the potential to be a genuinely transformative practice. Be courageous but gentle with yourself. Allow the gorgeous flow of trial and error as you take your first wobbly steps in this practice. Know that with practice will come both skill and wisdom.

LETTING GO AND GOING WITH THE FLOW

Relentlessly staying with the ongoing flow is essential to the practice. Skillful action is letting go of the stories you have accumulated about what sex and sexuality *should* look like, your stories of success and failure, and your confining goal-orientedness. If your deeply held belief is that sexual connection must always involve penetration, for example, then you are encouraged to notice how restricted that space is and do your best to let it go. Whatever you think "has to" happen obscures and numbs you to what is actually happening. This moment of sensual connection is always flowing forward. Be the flow.

The practice of going with the sensual flow is very much like the breath meditation practice, except that, rather than the breath, the focus of your attention will be the physical sensations of the unfolding present moment.

1. Begin the practice of going with the sensual flow in whatever way calls to you and your partner, however you would normally start sexual intimacy. For example, let's say that you start with kissing. In this practice, draw the present-moment attention that you have been cultivating in your

meditation practice to the physical sensations of kissing, allowing yourself to explore with curiosity and focused attention all the subtle sensations that are arising as though you are experiencing them for the first time.

2. As when you are following the breath, notice how the sensations are constantly shifting and changing from moment to moment. Notice, also, that your attention may wander to thoughts and judgments arising in your mind or to sounds and other sensations that are also present. When you notice that your attention has wandered away, gently and nonjudgmentally shepherd your attention back to the physical sensations arising from kissing.
3. Maintain this deliberate mindful attention to all the sensations that arise and shift as you continue exploring and deeply appreciating this unfolding moment of sexual connections between you and your partner.
4. Remind yourself that there is no goal involved in this practice except to vividly experience each passing moment of experience and to savor the sensations and connection between you and your partner. Intercourse is not the goal, though it may be something that happens. Orgasm is not the goal, though it may be something that happens. Whatever your ideas are of what should happen, simply notice their arising and allow them to bide their time and pass away without judgment, like leaves on a stream. Practice bringing your attention back to this unfolding moment and continue savoring the sensations of moment-to-moment touch.
5. Be especially attentive to moments when something that might have in the past been experienced as a failure occurs, because these are especially fruitful moments for letting go of expectations and returning your attention to the flow of what is actually happening. For example, if you or your partner loses an erection, practice gently accepting that as just another experience arising in the moment and flow forward to continue savoring and exploring what feels good and erotic. Remind yourself that the only goal is to savor and appreciate these few precious moments of sensual touch between you and your partner. There is no particular destination. Continue forward until either you or your partner is ready to move on, and then simply and gratefully move on.
6. Remember that you are committing only to presence and sensuality and to lovingly accepting whatever the moment brings. If your body cooperates with your intention, with erection, wetness, or opening, we accept that and flow forward. If your body does not provide erection, or wetness, or opening, accept that and flow forward into the next consensual erotic moment. If the sexual readiness of the body comes and goes, accept that and keep flowing forward. If things go as expected, accept that and keep

flowing forward. If things do not go as expected, embrace that and keep flowing forward.

7. Embrace whatever arises, and whatever arises is available to you in this moment of sexual connection.

How lucky and blessed are we to luxuriate in these human bodies?

Skillful, Generous, and Open

Through the lens of intimacy practice, the trio of sexual vitality is skillfulness, generosity, and openness.

Skillfulness is rooted in attention to your partner's sexual experience so that you can be a lifelong learner of what they find sexy, erotic, and sensual. Skillfulness, including being mindful of consent and boundaries, means paying loving attention and learning and feeling for what are this moment's turn-ons and turn-offs for your partner. It means staying open and present to the simple truth that we are both always changing and evolving and that what was a turn-on yesterday may be replaced by a slightly different turn-on today and by something newly lively tomorrow. Our sexual relationship is a vibrant, creative, and playful space. Skillful action is curious, attentive exploration of what is erotic and enlivening, following the path of the red thread to find out where it goes.

Generosity as a sexual intimacy practice means both knowing what is sexually exciting for your partner and acting on it. In our practice, it flows from lowering the barriers that separate us such that our partner's wants and desires are as palpable as our own. There might be things that your partner is really into that are basically erotically neutral for you (e.g., certain types of clothes or costumes, toys, or enacted fantasies), and the practice of generosity involves engaging in those things with joy and enthusiasm just because they bring your partner pleasure and joy. As long as engaging in the things that are sexually exciting to your partner does not diminish you or is not noxious or aversive to you, then their unique turn-ons become a gateway for the practice of sexual generosity, and the practice of sexual generosity is not only delightful but helps us to awaken from the illusion of separateness.

Our sexual relationship is a vibrant, creative, and playful space. Skillful action is curious, attentive exploration of what is erotic and enlivening.

Finally, the intimate practice of openness involves being attentive to our tendency to fall into sexual habits that no longer serve the cause of erotic connection. Though sexual patterns and rituals can serve an essential function in our intimate relationship—being both comforting and erotically evocative—staying squarely within the boundaries of the known and expected means that we may miss the opportunity to discover new sexual experience that we might find delicious.

Like a meal, sometimes we are in the mood for comfort food that we know will be delicious and satisfying, and sometimes we or our partner will be in the mood to try a dish, a flavor, a cuisine that we've never tried before. Love it or hate it, it is the newness and adventure, if entered with openness and joy, that matters. In your sexually intimate relationship, you might find that one of you is more naturally adventurous than the other, and the practice will be to create space for that difference and to be gentle and encouraging partners to each other as you openheartedly push into your growth edges.

Becoming a sexually skillful partner is rooted in the practice of mindful attention, which in turn helps us to see through the illusion of separateness and thus to embody an effortless generosity and nurture a deep trustworthiness that, in turn, makes us bold and adventurous. This is the practice of integration, wholeness, and awakening.

The Heart of the Matter

Any hope we have for intimate wholeness must include intimacy with our sexual nature—with mine, with yours, with all of ours. Great harm arises from disunion and separation. When I am separated from myself, I am dangerous to myself and others. When I am separated from others, I am dangerous to myself and them. Mindfully nurturing intimacy with our sexuality is essential to the path of awakening from the illusion of separateness. With the intention to be awake to our shared wholeness, with attention to the natural flow of the erotic through our lives, and with commitment to clarity and skillful action, we can rescue a sacred sexuality from a place of shame and confusion to take its rightful place as a gateway to intimate liberation.

This is what I have discovered: The practice of awakening from the illusion of separateness is sexy. It is vibrant. It is vivid. It is compelling. It draws us forward and blows us apart. It invites us to immersion and dissolution and union. It is the vitality of the unfolding of the infinite and unknowable. It is rich, earthy, sensual, ephemeral, gritty, lusty, and bright. As soon as we get a whiff of it, we are drawn to it. The Beloved. Take me with you. Envelop and enfold me. Free my yearning and desire. Give wing to every molecule of being. Blow it up. Burn it down. Build it back. Unfold me into the bright radiance of this brilliant precious life.

Mindful Mantra

As we enter this moment of intimacy, may we attune to one another.
When we are making love, may I be fully present,
May my touch bring you love, pleasure, joy, and passion.
May you feel safe and free enough in my embrace to come fully undone, knowing that I will be there to hold you.
May we give ourselves fully to each other—surrendering completely to the flow of the erotic.
May we remain endlessly curious about one another's ever-changing desires.
May our embrace dissolve the boundary that separates.
Opening our hearts fully, unguarded, may we take refuge in our longing and the free fall of our desire.
May the joy and fire of our union warm the world and set their spirits free.

PART III

OVERCOMING OBSTACLES ON THE PATH

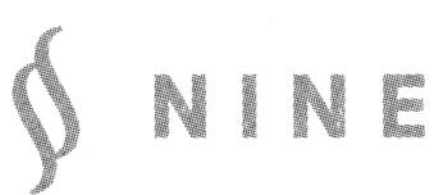

NINE

Burning Intimacy Bridges

PRACTICING WITH INTENSE EMOTIONS

First, we build intimacy bridges between each other's hearts. We seek acceptance, love, and safety, and we grant acceptance, love, and safety. We delightedly invite each other to shed our emotional armor. We each ask our partner to trust us with what is most vulnerable, with what is most easily wounded. And we promise to hold it all with love, care, tenderness, and respect.

Then, we burn those bridges down. Our beloved says or does something, or perhaps fails to say or do something, and we are cut and wounded. We deliberately ask for access to our partner's vulnerability but then disregard our responsibility to protect that vulnerability even when we are hurt. We seek to be close, but not too close. Close enough to feel a tiny bit of warmth, but not close enough to risk our hearts. Not again. As it turns out, when we cannot handle our own vulnerability, we will burn human connection to the ground to protect it. We are willing to destroy connection to protect our vulnerability, and we are left feeling lonely, hurt, and sick.

And so we react. Maybe by retreating into ourselves, withdrawing into our pain. Or maybe by lashing out—defending ourselves with angry words and actions. Anger in our relationships is always rooted in hurt, and we come by our reactivity naturally. The intensity of the emotion is real. It is understandable. It makes sense. But, when expressed completely indiscriminately, our words, at the mercy of a lifetime accumulation of hurt, can be incredibly harmful. We start to tear down the bridges we have built in an ill-fated and frantic attempt to protect ourselves.

In this chapter, I want us to turn toward the phenomenon of our emotional reactivity, our natural response to protecting our vulnerability. We'll learn ways to practice compassionate attention to our emotional reactivity in the service of deepening intimacy—even when every cell in our body is screaming to fight or run away. This is the courageous heart of the practice of wisdom and compassion. This is the path of intimacy.

Fight or Flight: The Fuel That Starts the Fire

As human beings, we inherit from our evolutionary ancestors only a small handful of instinctual reactions to pain, fight or flight being the most common. These primal responses to pain are hardwired in our nervous system, and by their nature are not reactions that we consciously choose or have the power to consciously choose not to experience. They are automatic. Fight responses function to chase away or destroy predators or rivals, for example. Flight responses function to get us out of dangerous situations as quickly as possible. These reactions are experienced in the body through the release of stress hormones, and they are often felt as heightened muscular tension, increased heart rate, faster breathing, and increased sweating. All of these physiological responses are designed to help us either physically fight or run away.

These automatic and natural reactions are not particularly helpful to us when the source of our pain is our partner's fussiness or unfolded laundry. In our relationships, if our partner does something that hurts our feelings or makes us mad, or if we get into an argument about household chores, or parenting, or sex, or in-laws, our body responds as though we are being physically attacked by an enemy or a bear. When we feel dismissed, rejected, criticized, or blamed, our most basic physical and psychological hardwiring responds as though we are under physical attack by an enemy.

When we follow the inner logic of fight or flight, we often end up snapping at our partner (name calling, criticizing, blaming, berating), or we break connection and run away (storming off, withdrawing, giving the cold shoulder). Unfortunately, these fight-or-flight reactions are much more likely to damage our intimacy than they are to resolve whatever the issue is. We are, mostly to our detriment, stuck with these ancient, primal, and destructive reactions in trying to nurture a modern, fragile, and complex intimate relationship.

When we feel dismissed, rejected, criticized, or blamed, our most basic physical and psychological hardwiring responds as though we are under physical attack by an enemy.

Some of the most interesting and impactful research in this area has been conducted by Dr. Janice Kiecolt-Glaser and her team at the Ohio State University College of Medicine. In a fascinating 1997 study in *Psychosomatic Medicine*, Dr. Kiecolt-Glaser and colleagues showed that even with newlywed couples who uniformly reported high relationship satisfaction, couples who expressed more fight behaviors, such as sarcasm, eye rolling, hostile tone of voice, and disgust, experienced increased stress hormone levels and, as a result, decreased immune system functioning, increased inflammation, and increased cardiovascular hazard markers (lower heart-rate variability). Even more interesting, in a follow-up study 10 years later in the *Journal of Consulting Clinical Psychology*, Dr. Kiecolt-Glaser and colleagues found that the stress hormones of these couples while they were still newlyweds were significantly higher in couples who later divorced or remained married in highly distressed relationships.

In other words, this and convincing related research has shown that couples more prone to unrestrained fight-or-flight responses are more likely to get sick, recover more slowly, heal from injury more slowly, experience more inflammatory diseases, age more quickly, and gain more weight, and they are more prone to depression.

All this is by way of revealing to us what we know about the physical and mental health damage that we experience when our emotional reactivity is acted out in unskillful and destructive ways. It is exactly this emotional reactivity that destroys intimacy, and most couples are completely at its mercy. We are enslaved to our emotional reactivity, and it inevitably pours gasoline on and ignites whatever intimacy bridges we have been lucky enough to build.

How can we put out the fire? Meet it with a spiritual practice of compassionately, mindfully attending to our emotional reactivity. This means learning to be intimate with our hurt, fear, and anger in the service of establishing, nurturing, and protecting intimacy.

Anger, the Gossamer Shield

We express anger hoping for healing, but instead get harm. Anger is one of the most destructive emotions in our relationships. It rises up as part of our fight-or-flight response to protect our vulnerability when we have been hurt. But it actually does a fairly lousy job of it. It is a shield made of gossamer. If you query your own experience, you'll see that even at your angriest, the deepest part of your experience is still pain and fear.

The best that the expression of anger can do is chase away the apparent source of our pain (or motivate others through their fear of us). In some cases, that is enough. We may remove the people in our lives who repeatedly cause us the most pain, and that may be the most skillful thing available to us. However, even in these cases, we still fully experience our hurt and vulnerability. So, in those relationships that we wish to preserve and protect, anger is only ever added to our hurt; it never replaces it. And yet, again, anger is our instinctual reaction, and it is precisely this reaction that we must turn to with love, attention, and kindness in our spiritual practice of intimacy.

We express anger hoping for healing, but instead get harm.

Researchers who have closely studied partners interacting with each other have repeatedly found that the most common response to anger is just more anger. When we express our anger unskillfully to our partner, it is virtually guaranteed that they will respond with their own expression of anger. If we yell, they will yell back. Or, if our partner is the more withdrawing type, they may go cold and silent, or simply walk away as a way of enacting their anger. In either case, like begets like.

John Gottman and colleagues, in their 1998 article in the *Journal of Marriage and the Family*, showed that what he calls a *hard startup* of an interaction becomes a kind of relationship gravity well, drawing everything else that happens in the conversation toward harshness. When we start angry, everything gets drawn toward anger. When we start with criticism, everything gets drawn toward criticism.

Anger is our instinctual reaction, and it is precisely this reaction that we must turn to with love, attention, and kindness in our spiritual practice of intimacy.

Alternatively, Gottman has also found that what he calls a *soft startup* has a similar gravitational effect, drawing the rest of the conversation toward softness. When we start with appreciation, everything gets drawn toward appreciation. When we start with compassion and empathy, everything gets drawn toward compassion. When we start with kindness, everything gets drawn toward kindness. Cause and effect can be both simple and relentless in their lawfulness.

So how do we, knowing the physics of relationships, take advantage of the opportunity provided to us by our own experience of anger so that we might wholeheartedly engage the practice of intimacy and relationship?

Setting the Intention to Receive Anger with Care

If we embrace the idea that everything that arises can be regarded as a gateway into the practice of intimacy, it holds for anger as well. Our experience of hurt and anger can lead us toward greater wholeness and actually heal our sense of separation and suffering. The setting of our intention, our vow as it were, is to turn toward our hurt and anger with loving attention and care, instead of simply acting out our anger in our typical reactive fashion. We vow to remain watchful for any instance of our experience of anger and recognize each such moment as an opportunity to enter the gateway into mindful intimacy practice.

I want to point out here that setting our intention is not yet actually doing the thing itself. The lived experience of it is that, if we're lucky, we notice our emotional reactivity, and we remind ourselves that our vow is to turn toward intimacy rather than to act out our reactivity. But, at this stage, all we may have is our intention. And that intention, all by itself, can be transformative.

In the study of forgiveness, we say that setting the intention to forgive is the essential first step on the path to forgiveness (see Chapter 13) *and* that it is not yet the experience of forgiveness itself. That experience emerges later, after we have been on the path for a while. Similarly, the intention to turn toward intimacy with our hurt and anger is the essential first step on the path to intimacy with hurt and anger. It is not yet the experience of intimacy with hurt and anger. Just being awake enough to remember our intention, however, is transformative.

We may wake up to remember our intention right in the middle of acting out our anger or withdrawal. We may be yelling or criticizing or angrily sulking when, through the grace of our ongoing dedicated meditation practice, we simply notice that we are yelling, criticizing, or angrily sulking. This moment of simply noticing changes everything. We may not yet be able to climb out of our hole. We may still be completely trapped in the tar pit of our angry withdrawal. We may still be dragged for some way by the momentum of flailing anger. But the noticing allows us to remember our vow, and remembering our vow allows us to reconnect with our intention to build and not destroy intimacy. This can be a life raft in a storm. It is our first step through the gate of practice right here, in the very midst of upset and reactivity.

Paying Attention to the Fire

When we catch ourselves experiencing the burn of hurt and anger, we enact our vow by first stopping whatever we're doing, dropping into our bodies, and rolling with the experience. Just like we were taught as kids to respond to catching fire: we stop, drop, and roll.

STOP, DROP, AND ROLL

Stop

Stopping means simply that you practice *refraining*. You catch yourself and simply refrain from acting out your anger in the same tired old pattern that has become your somewhat embarrassing lifelong habit. If you're yelling and cursing, or slamming, muttering, and stomping—just stop, notice what you're doing, take a deep breath, and bring yourself to stillness.

If you're in a car and noticing a moment of road rage, you might want to pull over, if it is safe to do so, or maybe simply settle into the stillness of the immediacy of driving the car. If you are at work or at home with your partner, and you are lucky enough to realize that you are experiencing and acting out your habitual anger dance, then it may be more available to simply stop what you are doing, breathe, and be still.

The great gift of stillness in such moments is that you immediately cease from adding any more harm to the moment—to yourself, to your partner, to your children, to the other drivers, to your coworkers, maybe even to the furniture. Maybe you find someplace to sit down, if you can. If your journal is handy, go to it and begin writing what you experience in the next two steps. Be still. Breathe.

Drop

Then draw your attention right here and drop into your body. Allow yourself to get really curious about where in your body you most palpably experience the presence of hurt and anger. Perhaps it is in your arms, chest, and jaw. Or in your forehead, eyes, and stomach. Where is it for you? Do you feel a tension and a tightening that feels like the precursors of fight and smash, tear and throw, stomp and slam, pound and punch? What do you feel yourself on the verge of?

You might then look even deeper, getting really curious to experience all of the nuances and fluctuations of sensation that make up that tension and tightening. Can you feel this as simply a kind of flow of sensation?

Roll

Then turn toward the sensations you associate with hurt and anger in the body and enact your vow to experience those sensations wholly, completely, and intimately, without turning away for even an instant. And then just breathe into that deeply intimate experience, without needing it to be any different than it actually is. You can say to yourself, "This is what it feels like. This is what is arising here. I can be with this. I don't have to do anything about it. I just have to notice and breathe. . . ."

As you sit, practicing intimacy with your anger, you will almost certainly discover that the roots of your anger are deep within your own hurt and suffering. That your anger is just a thick protective layer lying over your tender heart. That anger stands between your vulnerability and the world, trying its boct to chicld you from furthcr pain.

You can acknowledge with gratitude the fiercely compassionate bodyguard work of your anger. And then you can acknowledge and bring into the light your vulnerability. Practice by turning toward your tenderest places to discover the genuine strength within your undefended vulnerability. This is the fundamental discovery that awaits you—that it is your unwillingness to be vulnerable that makes you weak, brittle, and inflexible. When you can truly be intimate with your vulnerability, then you are always safely at home.

Take all the time you need to stay with the sensations of anger and vulnerability, looking deeply, concentrating, still, gentle, and caring. Maybe you can deliberately invite a small bit of relaxation into those muscles. If you can, that might feel quite wonderful, but it isn't necessary; it shouldn't be effortful or come from a place of harsh self-judgment. It should just be a small kind of letting go. And if the tension stays just as tense, that's also fine. Just looking deeply and breathing is enough.

After some time, you may begin to notice that the richness of the well-attended-to lived experience isn't really well captured by the simple words *hurt* or *anger.* What is actually happening is much too complex and lively for such a simple concept. This wild and vivid flow of energy simply is, like a stallion or a desert wind. And maybe it isn't really even ours. Maybe it is just something that is happening, like a hailstorm or a rainbow. Maybe this is just the universe unfolding in its own relentless and glorious way, as it has been doing from before the beginning. Maybe this is really all right, and just fine, and whole in and of itself.

What we might discover from this practice of mindful attention is that we are more than perfectly capable of sitting quietly with anger and hurt in its many forms, with the vulnerability we were born with and have accumulated. That serenity and equanimity are always with us.

And now that we have thoroughly entered the gateway of our anger to find our underlying tenderness, we can turn back toward the world, our beloved partner, our colleagues, our fellow drivers, and just do the next right thing—our best attempt to do the most good and the least harm. To do our own part in the ceaseless work of deepening our intimacy with ourselves, the world, and especially our beloved partner.

Skillful Action: Building Emotional Skillfulness

All the work of attention ultimately leads us to deeply consider what skillful action in the presence of hurt and anger is. I have both written about and conducted research on what I have come to call *emotional skillfulness.* Emotional skillfulness is precisely the practice of skillful action in the presence of strong emotions.

The field of psychology conceptualizes the experience of emotions in a range of ways, but the way that I find most helpful makes a clear distinction between the *internal experience* of an emotion such as hurt or anger and how we *behave* when we are experiencing that emotion. Psychologists tell us that we are always experiencing some type of emotion, regardless of whether we are aware of it or not. Our awareness of which emotion we are experiencing varies, because sometimes emotions are intense and obvious, and sometimes they are very subtle. In fact, we can think about the internal experience of any emotion as falling somewhere along two intersecting dimensions. One dimension goes from high intensity to low intensity, and the other dimension goes from negative to positive. So we can have high-intensity positive emotions, such as ecstasy, or low-intensity positive emotions, such as serenity. We can also have high-intensity negative emotions, such as rage, or low-intensity negative emotions, such as boredom. For our purposes in this chapter, we are mostly concerned with higher intensity emotion and emotions that are more negative. These are the emotions that we commonly think of as characterizing our emotional *reactivity*: anger, rage, jealousy, fear, panic, sadness, despair, loneliness, and so forth.

Our emotion *skills*, on the other hand, are the ways in which we've learned to behave in the context of any particular emotion. We can think of them as the behavioral repertoires that we have accumulated over the course of our lives as our own particular way of acting out our emotional experience. For example:

When we enact our *anger* as flight, we storm off, punishing the other with our absence and breaking connection. When we enact our anger as fight, we storm in and attack, punishing the other with our words and actions, and breaking connection.

When we enact our *loneliness* as flight, we withdraw and pout, saying nothing, but just signaling our hurt and upset. When we enact our loneliness as fight, we complain and criticize, punishing our partner for "making" us feel lonely, rather than inviting them to spend more time with us.

When we enact our *sadness* as flight, we shut down and pull away, pushing others away from us and cocooning ourselves in our despair. When we enact our sadness as fight, we get snappish and irritable, critical and difficult to please.

All of these ways of acting out our emotional experience are in some way attempts to escape our distress, trying somehow to make ourselves feel better. Unfortunately, more often than not, they don't work, and actually often only result in our feeling worse. In other words, they are unskillful.

Understandable, but unskillful.

So, on the one hand, we want to engage our mindfulness practice to begin to notice and name exactly what it is that we tend to *do* when we are feeling anger. On the other hand, we want to begin to notice whether what we do is actually *skillful* or not.

Does what you do build bridges (skillful action), or does it burn them down (unskillful action)?

Unfortunately, as I've noted previously, usually the form of our emotional reactivity, in its raw enactment of flight or fight, tends to do more harm to our intimacy than good. It makes us and our partners feel less safe, less secure, more separate and lonelier, and more distressed and disoriented. In other words, usually our emotional repertoire is quite. . . . unskillful. When we enact our hurt as anger, we obscure our tenderness and create division where there should be connection.

We want to notice what it is that we tend to *do* when we are feeling anger and whether what we do is actually *skillful*.

Having Anger Is Not a Choice

To be clear, strong emotions just happen. We don't choose them any more than we choose to catch a cold or get stung by a bee. They are automatic responses to our circumstances that flood our bodies and minds and that we find ourselves having to deal with, manage, and experience. Even the most experienced practitioner still experiences the arising of strong emotions such as anger, sadness, and fear. So we don't get to choose whether or not we have strong emotional reactions.

However, we can learn to practice intimacy with our strong emotional reactions such that we can develop ever more skillful ways of behaving in their presence. As we become more and more intimate with the lived experience of our strong reactive emotions, we become more and more familiar and comfortable with their presence. And, as we become more capable of simply being in the presence of our strong emotions, we open up the opportunity to practice more skillful ways of responding.

When we are angry, we can learn to behave in ways that are more likely to build connection and improve relationships. But, in order to do so, we must practice intimacy. We must practice turning toward our strong emotions, hosting them with gentleness and clarity. We must also practice turning toward others. Turning toward others with care and compassion. This is a challenging, difficult practice. But I believe that it is precisely this practice that is most necessary if we are to cultivate genuinely transformative relationships.

BEING EMOTIONALLY SKILLFUL

Let's look at how we might more skillfully enact our hurt and anger.

1. **Notice and acknowledge your own anger.** This simple and gentle acknowledgement—*anger is arising in me*—is key and crucial. It cuts through your inclination to lie to yourself about or simply deny your own emotional experience. It is an act of genuine self-compassion to acknowledge what is true in the moment. You can say to yourself, "I can feel anger arising and can acknowledge that I am not causing it, and neither is my partner. It is just gathering, like a storm cloud, and it is my responsibility to handle it with care. But I can only do so if I am honest and clear with myself that it is, indeed, here in my body and mind."
2. **Stop, drop, and roll.** Take adequate time to hold your anger close and gently care for it, until you know that you are safe, and it is safe, and everyone around you is safe. Whatever might need to be said or done, whatever might best serve the relationship, will still be true even if you give yourself hours to let your anger settle and soothe and your physiology return to baseline.

   Scientific studies have found that genuinely returning to physiological baseline can take up to 45 minutes. During this time, practice becoming intimate with all the sensations arising in your body and all the old and not so useful habit-pattern thinking in your mind. The more thoroughly you can give ourselves to the practice of deep and inquisitive allowing, the more you will grow in your capacity for equanimity and skillfulness.
3. **Respond skillfully.** Next, look to your partner and discern what the moment truly calls for. Sometimes it will be openhearted communication, and sometimes it will be something else, like self-care or stillness. The practice of skillful speech requires that we do our best to consider whether this is the right time to talk (or not). Is your partner available, do they have the time, and are they in the right frame of mind for what might be an emotionally challenging dialogue?

   Be mindful to say only what is most deeply true, to say only that which will heal and not harm, to speak gently with a loving tone, and to say only that which serves connection and intimacy. Skillful speech is an act of service for your beloved, not for yourself, but for connection, intimacy, love, compassion, nonseparation, and union.

   If your anger is hot and high, you might say something simple and descriptive like, *"I'm feeling pretty angry right now and I need some time to take good care of it. Thank you for being patient with me."*

If you have taken the time to settle, to touch your tenderheartedness, and the time is right to talk about it, you might first ask for consent to share, such as saying, *"I know that we still need to talk. I feel like I'm in a better place to do so. Is now a good time for you to continue our conversation?"* It is an act of great relational mindfulness to acknowledge that starting a conversation with your partner, especially one that might be difficult, is a request for their participation in something intimate, effortful, and resource consuming.

Clarify whether you are seeking emotional support or problem solving. You can say, *"I'm feeling sad and hurt. I don't really need us to solve that, I just want to share my experience with you and know that you care."* Or you might, for example, discover that your anger and frustration is rooted in loneliness and that loneliness needs a solution, for example: *"My love, I think I've been so fussy lately because I'm lonely. I miss you, and when work starts taking priority over us, it hurts my heart, and I respond with anger. Can we brainstorm ways that we can do a little more to put our relationship first?"*

4. **Engage in compassionate understanding.** Your foremost goal should be active listening in the service of your own compassionate understanding of your partner. Once you have thoroughly and empathically understood what it is like to be your partner, then your most skillful effort is to help your partner gain greater compassionate understanding of you. This practice can be especially challenging in the context of upset and anger, because in that moment what you most want to do is defend, complain, criticize, or lash out in some way. You are focused on your pain and are floundering to escape from it. In that moment, the lie inside the emotion is that the solution to your upset is to punish the other person, to make them feel as bad as you feel, to get them to admit fault, and to apologize, to make yourself feel better by asserting your dominance. The antidote to reactivity is empathy.

Empathy: The Antidote to Reactivity

It is radically emotionally counterintuitive to focus on empathic and compassionate understanding of our partner when everything in us is screaming for flight or fight. However, when we can prioritize wholly and empathically understanding what is going on inside our partner's heart and mind, then we know for certain that our intimacy practice is bearing real fruit. When we can both have and hold our own emotional stew and invite and receive the emotional stew of our partner, then we are actively participating in nonseparation. This is possible by actively engaging what I call our *empathic imagination*. It is an emotionally advanced skill, but essential for creating, nurturing, and maintaining true intimacy as a transformative practice.

> Mei was late coming home from work and hadn't called or texted. Steven was getting upset because he'd juggled all the after-work chores by himself, including starting dinner without any input or help, and he honestly felt a little taken for granted. He was genuinely getting more and more annoyed.
>
> And then he remembered the practice. He became aware of the growing anger in his body and mind, stopped what he was doing, and took a deep breath. He shifted his focus to intimacy with his experience and feeling for the tender spot that the anger was protecting. He noticed that he was tired, a little lonely and in need of a hug, and longing for food and rest and togetherness. He let that tenderness take its proper place.
>
> Then Steven used empathy and imagination to think about what might be going on for his partner. Maybe Mei was also tired, hungry, and in need of a hug. Maybe she had a stressful day that went too long and a stressful commute full of traffic. Maybe her mind was full of worry or upset about something he didn't even know about. Or maybe she got caught talking to a friend at work, really enjoying the conversation, and time got away from her. Maybe then she hit a streak of all her favorite songs and had been singing at the top of her lungs and just delighting in her drive home, genuinely not even imagining that she might be pushing some of his buttons.
>
> Steven made way for the arising of both compassion and sympathetic joy, so that he was as connected to any pleasure and joyfulness his partner may be experiencing as he was to any suffering she may be experiencing. When Mei finally walked in, Steven made room for the full blend of hard and soft emotions, and his feelings of care and concern about his partner, and then he greeted Mei with the tenderness that arises from knowing what a gift she is to him and how fragile they are in this world.
>
> Then, in the service of prioritizing compassionate understanding, Steven asked how her day was, how her commute was, and how she was feeling now. Once he felt connected to her experience and empathetic with what it is like to be her, he started to share his experience, how

his day had been, including that he was worried and upset that she was later than expected and hadn't called. Steven knew that he was practicing being skillful, and this helped to keep him mindful of his words and actions. He made sure that Mei knew that he didn't mean any harm. Then, looking to the future rather than correcting the past, he asked Mei to please try to remember to give him a heads-up next time she was running significantly later than usual.

Reclaiming Our Power to Connect

There is an enormous amount of freedom that comes from freeing ourselves from our habitually destructive reactive patterns. This also brings a very satisfying sense of relational competence, knowing that we are capable of shepherding this moment and our relationship toward connection, intimacy, and healing.

When, instead, we start with blame and shame, we actually give away our power to have a positive effect on our partner and our relationship, and we can end up feeling like we are at the mercy of forces outside of our control, including our partner's own reaction. But, as we've noted before, blame is almost always met with defensiveness, as our partner feels compelled to defend their integrity and good intentions; we just end up feeling invalidated and powerless to do anything but complain more bitterly. This move always ends in a lose–lose outcome.

If We're Lucky, It's Our Fault

The practice of intimacy begins with remembering our commitment to the path of awakening, with acknowledging our interconnectedness, and with the taking up of our responsibility for our own practice and our own relationship. If we are lucky, it's our fault. This is the practice of eating the blame.

There is a story in the Zen literature that goes something like this. One day at the monastery, the morning ceremonies ran long, cutting into the time the head chef had for preparing the noon meal. He hurried out into the garden to cut vegetables, and in his haste gathering vegetables, he cut off the head of a snake without realizing, and threw it in the pot with the rest of the soup. During the meal, the monks all said the soup was especially tasty, but the head teacher found something very interesting in his bowl. Holding up the head of a snake in his chopsticks, he demanded of the head chef, "What is this?" The head chef rushed forward, saying "Oh, thank you, Teacher!" and immediately grabbed the snake head, popped it in his mouth, and ate it.

There is an enormous amount of freedom that comes from freeing ourselves from our habitually destructive reactive patterns.

This is a story about our capacity to meet angry, painful moments in our relationship with absolutely no need to defend ourselves, but instead with the willingness and ability to respond with skill, care, and maybe even playfulness.

This story helps us to remember that our instinct to fight to make sure that nothing is our fault, more often than not, only serves to separate us from each other and to make whatever the situation is worse. The path of "it's not my fault" does not serve the cause of intimacy. This story also helps us to play with the possibility that not only might we be able to eat the blame with no harm but also that it might actually strengthen us and increase our capacity to take good and loving care of each other.

Eating the blame means freeing ourselves to respond to the moment in the most caring way possible. So, if we're lucky, it's our fault. Because then we can do something. If there is tension, then we can be the one who takes responsibility for moving more gracefully, more humbly, more skillfully to help both ourself and our partner steer toward more peaceful waters, more compassionate understanding, and deep connection. This is emotional skillfulness of the highest order, arising directly from our experience of genuine intimacy.

The Heart of the Matter

Intimacy is a lifelong practice. As we continue to swim in an ocean of openhearted vulnerability, we will regularly be blessed with opportunities to practice intimacy with our reactive emotions. So much of what ends up separating us from each other in our intimate relationships stems from the unskillful ways in which we react to the inevitable hurts, big and small, that occur when we are building an intimate relationship based on authenticity and vulnerability.

For many couples, genuine intimacy is simply too high a bar, simply too difficult to achieve in the absence of a dedicated intimacy practice. For many couples, "close, but not too close," a "good-enough" relationship, is truly good enough. But, for those of us who might aspire to engage in a truly transformative approach to intimate relationship, then this work of building, repairing, and maintaining intimacy bridges is essential. Our intimate relationships provide us with the perfect crucible for practicing with our most intense emotions, so that we might grow in the wisdom and compassion that saves us, saves our relationships, and saves all beings.

Mindful Mantra

May I turn toward pain and anger.
May I hold them close with love and grace.
May I allow them to rise and fall.
May I be curious about my partner's hurt and anger.
May I hold them close with love and grace.
May I allow them to rise and fall.
May I skillfully enact my hurt.
May I respond skillfully to my partner's hurt.
For intimacy and all beings.

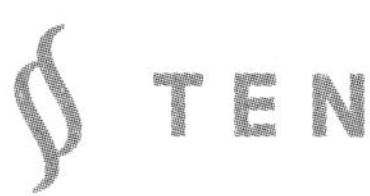

Awakening to Relationship Patterns

THE PRACTICE OF CO-CREATION

> **Awakening to our patterns allows us to love each other more artfully and transform our suffering into wisdom.**

We all fall into patterns in our relationships. These patterns are composed of the places where our vulnerabilities meet our partner's vulnerabilities—where our most fundamental differences get together to play—sometimes roughly. In this chapter, I introduce several of the most common relationship patterns that undermine intimacy and show you how you can transform these patterns into sources of playfulness and connection. You can use this chapter like a magazine quiz to identify the pattern traps that you and your partner tend to fall into. Awakening to our patterns allows us to love each other more artfully and transform our suffering into wisdom. My hope is that we can all find some humor, hope, and connection right in the midst of our most common human frailties, so that we might all wake up together to the joy of true intimacy.

Relationship Patterns Emerge

In our relationships, as part of this process of co-creation, some very common patterns emerge between partners. Some patterns serve our sense of partnership and connection, and others emerge as the habit patterns by which we enact our most common points of conflict. We discussed in a previous chapter the inescapability of perpetual issues. All couples, even the healthiest, will have at least a small handful of naturally occurring friction points between them that arise out of fundamental differences in personalities, temperaments, or learning histories.

What we know from the relationship science literature is that it is not necessarily the presence of perpetual issues that distinguishes healthy from unhealthy relationships; instead, it is the *quality* of the interaction that partners have concerning those issues. For example, the perpetual issue in your relationship might be that you react to stress by getting busy micromanaging all the worrisome little fires, and your partner reacts to stress by shutting down and avoiding as much as humanly possible. If you're lucky enough to stumble into a virtuous pattern, you might collaborate by using the ways in which your natural tendencies complement each other to help find the middle ground between fighting the stress and fleeing it. You support each other; there is union.

If, however, you fall into a destructive pattern, then you might find yourself in a perpetual tug-of-war, with you pulling toward getting things done and your beloved pulling toward putting things off. And this is what is often most characteristic of corrosive relationship patterns. One partner enacts their part of the pattern, and the other partner cannot help but react by enacting their opposing part of the pattern.

There are six destructive relationship patterns I most often see in my practice. Although these patterns ultimately aren't sustainable, they arise with goals that often are, such as to find calm, ensure safety, or experience joy. We might say that the intention of these patterns is well-being, but they wind up wreaking havoc on our intimacy. We'll go over each type and look at specific ways to break negative patterns. They are:

- The cactus and the fern
- The chef and the sous-chef
- The spender and the saver
- The porcupine and the turtle
- The introvert and the extrovert
- The mountain and the molehill

Once a reactive pattern has taken hold in a relationship, it can be virtually impossible to free oneself from it. Our patterns are so deeply ingrained that we cannot see them with any real clarity. When it is like this, our reactive patterns are in control; they are figuratively driving the bus, and we are just their long-suffering passengers, being driven through the same painful motions that we have been trapped in for as long as we can remember.

That which we are asleep to controls us.

So how do we wake up? By making a practice of breaking our poor habits and establishing skillful ones, that's how. Doing this, as you've been practicing in other chapters, involves three basic steps.

Step 1: Setting an intention. We simply allow ourselves to admit that we may be engaging in patterns that undermine our intimacy and then vow to become more aware.

Step 2: Paying attention. It is a relatively rare thing for partners to spontaneously wake up to their own patterns. But as our contemplative practice matures, we become better and better able to notice and articulate at least some of them. We practice noticing moments of conflict, then naming the pattern. This naming can serve as what Thich Nhat Hanh calls a "bell of mindfulness" for both partners. When we notice the pattern and can say with love and humor, "Hey, we're doing our spender–saver thing again!" then we are both instantly freed to try to meet the moment with more generosity and less constriction. Naming our patterns is an act of generosity. We also notice what's happening in our bodies; we become aware of the quality and content of speech and behaviors and their impact. This simple act of awareness changes everything. What once would have simply been an automatic and unexamined reaction becomes an opportunity to potentially do something more relationally skillful.

Step 3: Skillful action. We listen deeply to each other, we offer compassionate understanding of our partner's hopes and fears. With compassionate understanding, we will naturally cultivate a greater desire to collaborate toward mutually nurturing solutions that show that we care about each other's hopes and fears.

We review this process for each of the patterns. Keep in mind that both *inner work* and *relational work* must be done. The inner work is about finding the places within us where we are hooked by our own personal habits or our own unconscious reactivity. The relational work happens between us, where we can share our vulnerabilities and meet and hold our partner's vulnerability with acceptance and kindness. In this space of mutual vulnerability, we get to know each other more thoroughly; we form bonds of intimacy rooted in our common humanity and our genuine affection and compassion for each other.

The Cactus and the Fern

Goal: Affection and Space

I like to imagine that all of us fall somewhere on a continuum from desert plant to rain forest plant. In this metaphor, attention, affection, time together, and shared activities are the water that we all need to survive. The problem arises, then, when some of us require far more water than others.

In the case of the cactus and the fern, the partner who is naturally drawn toward more *interdependence*—closeness, time together, shared activities, lots of attention, and frequent affection—is the fern. They really only thrive in an atmosphere that is saturated with moisture. For fern people, a constant steady flow of attention, communication, affection, time together, and shared activities is essential for their optimal well-being. Ferns can tolerate periods of being alone, and may even desire it from time to time, but a little alone time goes a long way, and it is very easy for a fern to suffer terribly from dehydration. These partners are vulnerable to feelings of loneliness, separation, or abandonment.

The partner who is more naturally drawn toward more *independence*—individual pursuits, solo activities, alone time, less attention, and less frequent displays of affection—is the cactus. By their basic nature they need relatively little water to survive. In fact, it can be pretty easy to overwater a cactus, inadvertently killing it with misplaced kindness (ask me how I know this). Cactus people have a greater need for the direct sunshine of independence, alone time, and solo pursuits. They still need water—connection, affection, and time with their partner—even though a little goes a long way.

This partner is vulnerable to feelings of engulfment, encroachment, and being overwhelmed.

For some couples, the difference in need for time together versus time alone might be relatively small, but that difference can grow to be quite large under the right (or perhaps wrong) circumstances. As one partner starts to pull in the direction of more time apart (maybe spending more time engaged in a solo hobby), the other partner starts to pull harder in the direction of more time together (maybe wanting to add shopping together to the list of things they do as a team).

The partner who is more like a cactus, feeling a bit overwatered, might then pull even harder in the direction of alone time, maybe wanting to sit alone and read a book in the evening, rather than watching TV together. Pretty soon, through this type of polarization process, what might have initially been just a small difference can metastasize into a yawning chasm in which the cactus is always trying to get away to do solo things and the fern is always trying to get them to spend more time together. When this pattern is really in full swing, the cactus always feels a little too wet and the fern a little too dry, each resenting the other for their chronic discomfort.

Intention, Attention, and Skillful Action with the Cactus and the Fern

As always, begin by setting an intention. You must decide that both affection and space are necessary for survival, and that too much or too little water can be destructive. So you set an intention to be willing to build awareness, assess the pattern, and take steps toward more intimacy.

The next step is paying attention. With growing awareness, you might notice that whenever your partner pulls in the direction of more togetherness, your mind pulls in the direction of time alone. Or you might notice that whenever you pull in the direction of time alone, your partner reacts by seeking more time together. Notice this pattern without too much judgment and reactivity, as a kind of force of nature, like when the wind blows, the trees sway, or the stars shine through when the sun sets.

So, with attention, become more intimately familiar with what the arising of a cactus reaction or a fern reaction feels like in your body. Where is the tension? Do you feel yourself pulling against your partner in the direction of greater autonomy? Simply allow that tension and make room for it in your experience. Or perhaps you feel your body and heart constrict when you feel the tug of your partner pulling toward independent action. Breathe into it and open up some spaciousness. Give yourself permission to just feel the way that you feel without having to do anything about it or make it do anything different.

As mentioned throughout this book, so much of what drives us to destructive words and actions arises from our inability to simply tolerate our own discomfort. So much of what frees us from the prison of our own reactivity arises from our growing intimacy with the raw experience of our simple discomfort.

Also notice the habitual thoughts that arise in the mind. Maybe, as a cactus, they are thoughts about how you "never have any time" or how you don't get to do enough of your own things. Maybe you want to be able to visit friends, or go to particular stores, or watch the shows that only you are interested in. It really could be anything that you feel fussy about needing your own independent time to do. Or maybe, as the fern, you have repetitive thoughts about not feeling prioritized, cared about, or wanted. Can you simply watch those thoughts arise and give them space?

Noticing our habitual thoughts without being entranced by them is one of the most important fruits of intimacy practice. We want to slowly accumulate the ability to simply notice the arising and presence of our thoughts without necessarily believing them and living inside of them. We are capable of simply noticing our thoughts as thoughts, and with this we are freed to determine whether those thoughts are beneficial to our connectedness with the world or not.

Next, you can name the pattern aloud. In this way, you are able to shift out of tug-of-war mode and into both–and mode. The more you are able to call your pattern by its name, the less you'll engage in that pattern. Rather than seeing the day as a competition between interdependence and independence needs, you can see it as an opportunity to make sure that you are, together, taking good and loving care of each other. We get to live lives of generosity and care, rather than stinginess and defensiveness.

Finally, you can begin to practice the trial-and-error search for more skillful action. So, for example, in the presence of the thought, "what about me?" you might simply notice that thought and the constrictions that accompany it, holding it with great warmth and tolerance, and then choose to be collaborative with your partner, rather than competitive. You might say, "Hey, sweetie, let's figure out how we're going to spend our day. I'd like to spend some quality time with you, and I'd also like to go for a long run by myself. How about you?"

If you are a cactus-and-fern couple, I invite you to be grateful for your pattern.
It's a gateway to intimacy if you will only enter it.
May you know both sunshine and rain in equal measures, and may you be a source of love and care for each other for all of your days.

The Chef and the Sous-Chef

Goal: Coping with Anxiety

The chef and the sous-chef pattern is about power—exerting power or escaping power to cope with anxiety. In general, this pattern is characterized as one in which one partner has emerged as the de facto supreme manager in the relationship and the other partner has emerged as the assistant to the manager. We can name this pattern in many ways. Sometimes we call it the boss and the employee pattern, or the teacher and the student, or the expert and the novice, depending on the particular dynamics at work in the relationship.

For example, it is not uncommon for this pattern to arise quite naturally in a couple's parenting relationship. When partners first start out as parents with their first child, both start out on equal footing, knowing almost nothing about how to effectively care for this particular child.

However, at some point, at least one of the parents inevitably must go back to work. During that first Monday back at work, the parent who stays home gains 8 to 10 hours of more hands-on training in effective baby care. By the time the other parent returns from work, that parent is already at least a little bit behind the curve in terms of knowing what is working for their baby today. Slowly but surely, one parent emerges as the more practiced and expert parent, and the other parent becomes the parent who helps the expert. Now there is a power differential.

The expert parent has become the one in charge, and the novice parent has become the one following instructions. Even when something happens that is a new challenge for both parents, such as the first time the baby gets sick, the newly expert parent will step forward to take over, even though they also have never taken care of a sick baby. The pattern has taken over.

With this pattern comes a whole host of very predictable resentments. The expert parent becomes increasingly resentful that the more novice parent isn't doing as much to help and can't seem to get it quite right. The novice parent begins to feel like every attempt to step up is being carefully observed by the other partner, who is anxiously waiting to take over. The expert parent becomes increasingly frustrated with the sense that *if it's going to be done well, I'll just have to do it myself.* Both parents become exhausted, feeling unappreciated, overburdened, irritated, resentful, and confused. This pattern can leave both partners feeling incredibly lonely.

It should be noted that this pattern is the exact opposite of sexy. This expert–novice pattern is often the fissure through which all sexual chemistry and desire seeps out of the relationship. It is difficult to feel sexually attracted to someone who is giving you marching orders and quick to point out your failures. It is equally difficult to feel sexually attracted to someone who you resent for making your life harder rather than easier.

Another feature of the power imbalance is that we often have a hard time giving it up. The expert parent might be overburdened, but they get the comfort of the certainty that they are the last word on all things parenting related. The novice, on the other hand, might feel bossed around, but they get to focus on other things without feeling the overwhelming responsibility of being the one who is ultimately in charge of the child. Both partners are always losing, but both partners are also always winning. And it is this dialectic that makes this pattern so difficult to free oneself from.

The chef–sous-chef pattern can emerge in almost any area of our relationships. Whatever the domain, the pattern takes the form in which there can only be one chef in the kitchen, and there is only one right way to make a soufflé and load a dishwasher. The sous-chef can help, but they don't get to make independent decisions and must always work under supervision.

For those couples who wish to free themselves from this pattern, we are looking for a new way of being in which there is greater role flexibility and shared expertise. We are aiming for a relationship in which both partners are comfortable taking the role of chef, and both partners are equally comfortable taking the role of sous-chef. We call this "step forward–step back."

Intention, Attention, and Skillful Action with the Chef–Sous-Chef Pattern

Begin by setting your intention. Having become aware of a chef–sous-chef pattern in your relationship, you must first decide that it is doing more harm than good and that you are willing to give up the benefits of your role in the pattern to practice stepping forward and stepping back. The question to ask yourself is, "Is there a domain of my relationship where one of us almost always has the final say, sets the standard, or calls the shots?" It can be about big decisions, such as where you both will live and whose job takes precedence. It can involve who makes decisions about the house—which projects are a priority and how things should look and be. It can involve who decides what's for dinner. Or it can involve how the family finances are handled. Bring awareness to that area in your life and make a vow to practice mindful attention around it.

The next step is to harness your attention. If you are often stuck in the chef role, start noticing when you are assuming the lead in certain situations. Are you assuming ultimate authority for parenting? What are you worried might happen if you weren't always vigilant and in charge? What would it feel like to have another chef in the parenting kitchen who does things differently from you? Maybe they handle bedtime with more or less flexibility? Maybe they respond faster or slower to sounds of distress from the baby? Maybe they make doctors' appointments right away, or maybe they procrastinate? Maybe they hover in the playground, or maybe they hang way back? What is it like to encounter their difference and to feel the discomfort arise in your body? Can you breathe into that discomfort and invite some spaciousness within which discomfort can simply be, without necessarily doing anything about it?

If you are stuck in the sous-chef role, notice when you find yourself stepping back and letting your partner take control. Notice what is happening in your body and your mind when you pass responsibility on to your partner. Do you feel relief? Do you feel guilty? Do you feel freed? Whatever it is, make a note of it. Find where it lives in your body and breathe into it, making space for that feeling without having to change it.

For the sous-chef, imagine stepping forward and assuming full responsibility for some of the facets of parenting. Does it feel scary? Does it feel overwhelming? Do you feel incompetent? Do you just wish someone else would do it for you? Whatever those feelings are, just notice them and try to invite some kindness and grace. You might say, "I guess I do feel scared of being in charge and relieved when my partner takes over. That's okay. That's real. No judgment. I can feel this way and still step forward, rather than reactively stepping back." Now it's time for skillful action. As the chef, when you notice yourself clinging to control, you can say, "I'm doing my chef thing again." This, in and of itself, has the power to change the dynamic, giving you room to potentially try something new, to step back and let the other partner assume control. You might talk with your partner about creative ways to challenge the pattern, such as taking turns with being in charge of mornings or evenings. You might say, "I'll be the parenting chef when it comes to doctors' appointments, and you'll be the parenting chef when it comes to communicating with the school."

One of the biggest challenges for the chef is letting go of power and control. Power and control are often rooted in fear. The thinking goes, "When I am in control, I am safe. When someone else is in control, I feel scared." Giving up power and control does not come naturally to the chef, so it must be practiced.

Skillful action from the perspective of the sous-chef is challenging, because it requires you to assume control even though you're afraid that you'll blow it, make mistakes, or fall short in some way. Instead, talk to your partner about taking over responsibility for aspects of your shared parenting. Maybe you can play with an idea such as "Parent of the Day." Parent of the Day makes all the important calls on that day, and the other parent assists. "I'm Parent of the Day on Mondays and you're Parent of the Day on Tuesdays." Or you can divvy up domains of responsibility, such as homework versus extracurriculars or breakfast versus dinner. Allow yourself room to learn by doing. This will mean embracing the trial-and-error process necessary for becoming an expert chef. Sometimes the soufflé will fall. Sometimes the doctor's appointment will be missed, or bedtime won't go so smoothly. That's good. We learn by failing and trying again.

The same basic advice holds regardless of where in your relationship you manifest the expert–novice pattern. If it's about money, what is it like to loosen your grasp on the reins of control or to step forward and assume control and responsibility? If it's about the house and home, what's it like to let your partner load the dishwasher their way or to take responsibility for keeping the kitchen clean? Whatever it is, notice where you reactively grab control and practice letting go, or where you reactively flee from responsibility and practice stepping forward and assuming the lead.

May all of you who are caught in the painful pattern of chef–sous-chef find your way to shared expertise and shared incompetence.
May you know the joys of your different ways of doing things.
May you revel in your ability to step forward and step back in equal measures.
May you, your children, and all beings benefit from your practice.

The Spender and the Saver

Goal: Safety and Joy

The spender–saver pattern is easily one of the most common patterns that couples fall into. For the person who is on the more extreme end of the saver continuum, there is nothing more virtuous and comforting than saving money and having money safely tucked away; spending money, even when absolutely necessary, is always at least a little bit painful. For the person who is on the more extreme end of the spender continuum, the main point of having money is to spend it on the things we need and want; there is nothing more wonderful than spending hard-earned money to make our lives better and enjoy what is here to be enjoyed right now.

All of us fall somewhere on the spender–saver continuum. However, even a small initial difference can ultimately polarize into a large and painful area of conflict. If we are just a little bit more of a saver than our partner, there will come a time when their spending is just a little too rich for our comfort, and we'll find ourselves reacting by doing something to protect how much we are saving. We may tell our partner to slow down on the spending. Or we might start taking peanut butter and jelly sandwiches to work in an effort to offset our partner's spending. In other words, when something our partner does pushes on our saver button, we react by pulling harder in the direction of saving.

Similarly, if we are a little bit more of a spender, there will come a time when our partner's impulse not to spend money will feel just a little too stingy, and we'll react by making sure that we aren't depriving ourselves of the things we need or of the joy of just getting something that we want. We might spend money against our partner's will, feeling justified because it's money we earned. In other words, when our partner does something that pushes our spender button, we react by pulling harder in the direction of spending more.

For the saver, day-to-day life is like walking a tightrope strung between two skyscrapers, and money is the safety net. The more savings they have, the safer they feel. Working hard to weave more money into the net provides insurance against the many things that can, and often do, go wrong. Until they feel that their safety net is sufficient to catch and hold their weight, they simply cannot feel safe.

For the spender, it's as though they have lived too many years inside a small cell, deprived of all the joys that life has to offer. Now that they are free, they are determined not to suffer deprivation again. They are committed to living a life in which they work to live and are suffocated by the thought of living to work. For spenders, money is about being able to celebrate life, and not being able to use money to celebrate the richness of life feels like being shoved back into that old, cold cell. They don't want to deprive themselves and the people they love of the things money can buy just to squirrel it away for some rainy day that may never come.

Intention, Attention, and Skillful Action with the Spender–Saver Pattern

Setting our intention to practice intimacy with the spender–saver pattern means encouraging our willingness to turn toward the emotional pain at the heart of habitual reactions about money. As with so many domains of practice, this is often so much easier said than done. Our emotional relationship with money is often thoroughly rooted and tied to some of our deepest hurts and fears. So setting this intention is, in and of itself, a true act of courage.

You can say, "Whatever arises, I vow to turn toward it, to hold it close and gently, hosting it with generosity and kindness. I will refrain from the things I usually say and do and, instead, inviting stillness, I drop into my body to get to know how it is feeling and responding."

Having spent some time looking deeply into the physical sensations, you might then turn your attention to the thoughts that are arising in your mind. Notice their patterned nature and how they are so often the same thoughts on repeat. Are they thoughts of victimhood, of unfairness, of right and wrong? What emotions and impulses do each of those thoughts create? Do they make you want to strike out or say hurtful things? Do they make you want to withdraw and go quiet, turning away from your partner and into resentment and blame? Noticing the thoughts as thoughts can release us from their tight grip, even if it doesn't necessarily erase them from our minds. Noticing the impulses that arise from those thoughts can unhook us from their automatic nature, so that we might refrain from simply mindlessly enacting them yet again.

Finally, you can turn toward any action that serves the loving connection between you and your partner. This almost always begins with empathy and doing your best to feel your way into your partner's experience. This requires the humility to let go of your own perspective and agenda, temporarily but completely, so that you might focus entirely on the project of compassionate understanding.

Knowing how important spending or saving is to your partner, be kind and helpful, and find a way forward that serves you both. Maybe, when you have an extra $100, you decide to save half and spend half. You might decide that $50 goes to the safety net, and $50 is spent in the service of abundance and vibrancy. This is perhaps overly simplistic as an example, but it communicates the spirit of generosity and giving from a place of care and kindness that should exemplify skillful action in relation to the spender–saver pattern.

If your partner is prone to hesitating on a purchase because of a saver impulse, you can say, "OK, sweetie—we don't have to make a decision today, let's go home and sleep on it," or, at times, "Love, you work so hard, and you've been wanting this for a long time, I think it could be really wonderful if you let yourself buy it."

To highlight the spiritual practice here, you set your sights on cultivating intimacy with both yourself and your partner. Assess how you can become more intimate with your own habits and reactivities regarding money. Look at how you continuously nurture greater intimacy with your partner through the vehicle of spending and saving. Take up this practice to free yourself from the illusion of separateness, so that you can know your own wholeness and create an intimacy refuge for your partner and yourself.

May all the spender–saver couples out there know that you are safe and know that you are free.

May you find balance in the difference of your natures.
May you acknowledge how your life and history shape your relationship with money, and may you compassionately move toward greater harmony, for you, your partner, and your shared dreams.

The Porcupine and the Turtle

Goal: Relief and Connection

The porcupine and the turtle pattern describes partners who react to the stress of conflict in very different ways: either through flight or through fight. That is, one partner is compelled to pursue on the offensive (the porcupine, who protects its vulnerability through sharp measures), whereas the other partner is equally compelled to withdraw on the defensive (the turtle, who seeks protection from further harm within its shell). It is a pattern that can be very painful for both partners and can lead to a great deal of frustration and resentment.

When conflict arises, one partner might react by pulling back a little bit, tucking their head just an inch or so into their shell. The other partner, sensing their withdrawal, might react by pursuing, asking "What's wrong?" Feeling the tension escalating, the turtle then pulls even further into their shell. The porcupine partner then pursues further, quills out, trying to get the conflict out in the open where it can be dealt with. Ultimately, the porcupine finds themself on the outside of their partner's shell, fighting hard to get them to come out, and the turtle finds themself feeling overwhelmed, simply weathering the quill storm until it's over.

One of the things to keep in mind is that both styles are after the same thing: relief and connection. For the turtle, the best ways to experience relief are to avoid conflict in the first place or to withdraw and wait for the storm to pass. For the porcupine, the fastest and most efficient path to relief is through airing out the conflict and resolving it.

Unfortunately, both partners' underlying assumptions about conflict are wrong. Within the porcupine's attack is an unexamined assumption that fighting will lead to winning, and winning will lead to peace. I've always found it mysterious and disheartening that inside our urge to fight is the false promise that we can crush our way to feeling better. The more aggressively we fight, the more damage we do, the more conflict we experience, the more harm we experience, and the more bridges we burn with the very people who might otherwise be sources of love and support.

Similarly, within the turtle's withdrawal is the assumption that all sources of tension will simply resolve themselves if we just refrain from making them worse. However, unrelenting conflict avoidance always leaves resolvable issues unresolved. Withdrawal doesn't even really avoid conflict. Instead, it transforms conflict into something more passive and muddier. We end up signaling our unhappiness rather than talking clearly about it. Eventually, the pattern can burn itself and the relationship out. The porcupine will simply stop trying to get through the turtle's shell and start to turn away from the relationship. The turtle will mistakenly think that the relationship has suddenly healed itself, taking the absence of conflict as a sign that everything is better now, rather than recognizing it as the death knell of the relationship itself. This is why it is vitally important for couples to recognize when they are stuck in this pattern, so that they might free themselves from it before it corrodes the foundation of their intimacy.

Intention, Attention, and Skillful Action with the Porcupine–Turtle Pattern

When the impulse to fight arises, we fight. When the impulse to flee arises, we flee. Even if those impulses are suppressed, we still find ways to express them through either passive aggression or passive flight. So you start here, by simply acknowledging that these are powerful physiological forces that are not easily befriended. Set an intention to turn toward moments of intense fight-or-flight impulses with intimacy, equanimity, care, courage, and kindness. Set your sights on the North Star of more skillfully loving your partner by being able to leap free of your pattern, though you know the journey may be long and challenging.

Next, you can start to bring your practice of attention to moments when you and your partner are caught in our porcupine–turtle pattern. Practice noticing what you are doing, seeing what is unfolding between you both, and choosing, on purpose, to either continue your pattern or to try something more in keeping with your intimate intent and your values.

Then, simply name what you are noticing. You might say, "Oh, wow, I am really withdrawing hard right now. We must be doing our porcupine–turtle pattern." Or "I just want to yell and scream and say hurtful things. I'm feeling angry. I'm acting the porcupine here. I'm going to sit with this feeling a moment, nonjudgmentally, even as I feel desperate to act out."

You can turn toward your partner and practice empathy and deep listening. Maybe say, "I don't like being turned away from you, and I want to try turning back and reconnecting. I know that my turning away hurts you and that you are upset about something that genuinely matters. I want to try to understand better. I only ask that you please try to be careful with my feelings while you are helping me to understand."

Or, "I don't like feeling like I am fighting you. I want to stop pushing and just do my best to understand and connect. I know it hurts you when I just complain and criticize. I know you want to stay turned away from me right now, and I don't know how to help you feel safe to come out of your shell. Just know that I am here, and I am ready to listen when you are ready to come out and share with me."

If your partner does respond to your invitation (and being inviting is key), then you are gifted with the opportunity to practice receiving feedback with humility and without defensiveness. What your partner is describing about their experience is genuinely and undeniably their experience. It may not be perfectly worded. It may feel full of inaccuracies and unbalanced blame. It may feel unfair and biased. It may be all these things and more, and even so it is a gift because they are taking the risk of sharing with you their genuine experience.

When you can receive them graciously, then, and only then, can you richly engage in the practice of relating to each other authentically. You can show your partner that you heard them by simply offering back, without judgment, something like this: "It feels to you like you are doing mostly everything, and even though you acknowledge that I also work hard, it still seems like the lion's share of the scut work falls on you, and it is hard and lonely work, and you just wish that I was there for more of it. Is that right?"

Then you can apologize for having contributed to their pain. You might say, "I'm so sorry for what I have done and what I failed to do that has made you feel burdened and alone. I don't want that for you. I want us to find a way to do this that feels more equitable and connected."

Finally, if necessary, you might choose to share your experience more vulnerably so that your partner might also know you better. You might say, "When you leave things undone or messy, I want to assume that you had an understandable reason—that you were busy or got distracted or even just didn't have the energy to get it done. I see that you work hard all the time and are not lazy or negligent. Then I either straighten it up myself or maybe also choose to leave it for now. I'm worried that when you see that I have left something undone or messy that I am not getting a similar kind of benefit of the doubt. It scares me that you might be assuming, even unconsciously, that I am lazy, or thoughtless, or carelessly sexist. I think that's why I have such a strong reaction when you call me out about clutter in the house."

MOVING TOWARD RELIEF AND CONNECTION

Having encouraged yourself to come out of your shell or to stop fighting, you can:

1. Prioritize understanding your partner's experience.
2. Take responsibility for what you have done, even accidentally, that has caused your partner pain.
3. Vow to do better now that you know better.
4. Risk the vulnerability of sharing your own experience, perception, delusion, and field of thoughts, both rational and irrational, entrusting your self into the care of your beloved.

None of us come out of the box with all the skills that we need to build intimacy and connection out of our porcupine–turtle pattern. The key is committing ourselves to the trial-and-error of an ongoing relational practice, a spiritual practice out of which we forge deeper intimacy and greater wisdom and reconnect with our inherent wholeness.

May all of the porcupines and turtles stay present and be gentle with each other.
May you practice venturing outside of your instinctual comfort zones in the service of great connection.
May you take great care to love each other with your quills down and your heart out.
May you delight in the different creature you fell in love with and stay curious about what makes them move in the world.

The Introvert and the Extrovert

Goal: Recharging

For whatever weird quirk of nature, introverts and extroverts can't keep their hands off each other and end up partnering up in droves. Maybe introverts are attracted to the sociability and excitement extroverts exert in their element. Similarly, for extroverts, winning the attention and affection of an introvert can feel like a rare gem. However, even a small difference on this continuum can create the conditions for polarization and conflict.

The introvert–extrovert pattern often plays itself out when both partners are tired and each just wants to recover from their exhaustion. For example, it might be Friday night, and both partners are tired and stressed from a long week juggling all the demands of work and family. The extrovert just wants to go out and be around people and do something fun, and the introvert just wants to put on their pajamas, sit on the couch, and binge-watch movies.

Intention, Attention, and Skillful Action with the Introvert and Extrovert Pattern

Begin by making a promise to notice that this pattern exists in the first place. You can say, "I can relate to the introvert–extrovert pattern, and I'm vowing to pay more attention when I see it unfolding. I want more connection with my partner, and working on this pattern is going to help."

The next key to compassionately understanding the introvert–extrovert pattern is simply noticing and naming it—such as, "Gosh, my partner always wants to go out, and I just hate it. I'm tired and overwhelmed and just want to relax." Or, "Gosh, my partner only ever wants to stay home and watch TV, and I just hate it. I want to go out and enjoy my time off." Noticing these types of thoughts is the first clue that you are probably in the grip of the introvert–extrovert pattern.

Naming the conflict as a *pattern* puts the blame onto the pattern, rather than your partner. When the blame goes to the pattern, then you and your partner are once again on the same side of things.

Then, for this pattern in particular, the key is developing mutually compassionate understanding for each other. The extrovert and introvert personalities appear to be deeply baked into us, often genetically, and it is not a choice or habit that can simply be changed. You are who you are—introvert or extrovert. So you acknowledge that this is simply how you are hardwired, and that is simply how your partner is hardwired.

The challenge of perception is that it can be hard for partners to clearly see this difference in each other. Introverts can appear to be quite extroverted. In fact, lots of people who are comfortable performing in front of audiences are actually introverts by nature. Introverts can also be gregarious and know how to expertly work a room. Similarly, some people who spend a lot of time in solitary professions are actually extroverts by nature. Extroverts can work as coders or writers, spending hours working by themselves.

So it isn't necessarily the way we present in our day-to-day lives that categorizes us as more introverted or more extroverted. Instead, it is in how we plug in and recharge that reveals our fundamental introvert–extrovert nature. If you are a classic introvert, when your battery is blinking red, you recharge by spending time alone or with just the few people in your bubble, if you will. Similarly, extroverts recharge by being around others; it is the social buzz that refills their energy stores. After a long day of exhausting work, nothing does the trick quite so well as going out with friends and socializing for a while.

Once we realize that we are both after the same goal—recharging—then we are in a much better place to collaborate and care well for each other. You can say, "I know we are both tired and need to recharge. Maybe after dinner I can go out to play volleyball with my friends while you watch some TV, and then we can hang out together when I get back? What do you think?"

When you can see and feel that your partner cares as much about your happiness and well-being as their own, then you learn at a bone-deep level that you can trust them with what is most vulnerable and true. This is how you build an intimate home for each other using the very material of the introvert–extrovert pattern that you used to struggle with.

May all introverts and extroverts come to love their true nature.
With compassion and wisdom may you help each other to rest and recharge.
May you know that in the end you are not two batteries, but only just this one—shared to brighten the world and help all beings.

The Mountain and the Molehill

Goal: Calm

The mountain–molehill pattern arises between partners out of a naturally occurring difference in how they each respond to acute stressors. For some of us, when something stressful happens, we want to be able to take it in stride, place it in its proper context, fit it into the overall priority list, and then just do whatever is necessary to address the issue in the least stressful or bothersome way possible. For others of us, when something stressful happens, we want to be able to address and resolve it as quickly as possible and to give it all the attention that we think it deserves, even if that means putting as much as possible aside so we can dedicate our attention to dealing with the issue at hand quickly. Both approaches can be quite practical, and each works in its own way to effectively resolve most issues. The trouble of the pattern arises when each partner starts to react to how the other partner naturally responds to a crisis.

For example, let's say the check-engine light goes on in the car. One partner's instinct might be, "Shoot, I don't have time to deal with that right now. I'm sure it'll be fine until this weekend when I can get it into the shop. I'll call the mechanic when I get to work and see when getting it in fits in my schedule." The other partner's instinct might be, "Shoot, I need this car to not give out on me. I'm going to have to cancel my afternoon meetings and see if I can get into the mechanic today before it gets any worse."

These two responses are all well and good if one or the other partner is in the car alone when this happens. However, if they are both in the car at the same time, then the mountain–molehill pattern is almost guaranteed to arise. The mountain partner starts to feel more anxious because the molehill partner doesn't seem to be taking the problem seriously enough. They then raise the emotional stakes to try to impress on the other partner the urgency of the situation, such as saying, "I don't think we can wait until the weekend. What if it's something serious? I need you to take this seriously." The other partner, feeling increasingly stressed by their partner's response, might try even harder to minimize the urgency of the situation while defending themself against the implied criticism, for instance, "I am taking it seriously, but honestly, I don't know why you have to panic about these things. It isn't a big deal. It can wait a few days. Don't worry about it."

Well, as you know, the phrase "don't worry about it" has never in the history of intimate relationships actually worked as intended. It is the equally ineffective cousin of "calm down."

Intention, Attention, and Skillful Action with the Mountain-Molehill Pattern

Starting with an intention to see and name this pattern has a power all its own. However, an important piece with this pattern is to commit to cultivating a growing sense of humility and to take ourselves lightly. As the burden of your fear-driven concern to protect your own ego diminishes, you are better and better able to meet these moments of pattern recognition with humor and generosity.

Rather than feeling threatened or called out when you or your partner names the pattern, can you instead feel deeply amused? Amused with the same warmth and relief that you feel when you find your missing glasses waiting patiently for you right on top of your head? You might respond, "Oh, we're doing our pattern again. Isn't that funny? Isn't that just so us?" If you're prone to making an issue a molehill, you can chuckle, "Okay, I'll stop molehilling. I don't want you to miss your important meeting this afternoon, but I do have some less important things I can move around tomorrow if the mechanic can take it then. Would you be comfortable waiting just one more day?" If you're prone to making an issue a mountain, you can say affectionately, "Yeah, I don't want you to have to drop everything. I think it'll be okay until tomorrow. Thank you for taking it on. That really makes me feel cared for."

Intimacy practice calls on you to recognize and hold each other's tenderness and vulnerability with ceaseless care and clarity. The paradox is that, rather than this making you more fragile, it actually makes you stronger and more resilient to the slings and arrows that are a natural part of what it means to be a human being. You are doing your very best. Your heart is in the right place. Your deepest nature is compassion and union. There is strength in vulnerability, and our practice is the path to freedom.

May the mountain and the molehill see their reflection in each other and know that they are not separate.

May you find humor and cheer in your differences and gladly gaze upon the world through your partner's lenses.

May you join in the space between molehill and mountain, where the flowers and the grasses point the way.

The Heart of the Matter

In truth, we continually co-create each other. Everyone that we encounter changes us. We, in turn, change everyone we encounter. And there is no place where this is more powerfully true than in our closest, most intimate relationships. We create and are created by each moment that unfolds between us. We are who and what we are in this moment, arising out of our mutual entanglement with our partner. Our partner is who they are and what they do because of the blending of their unfolding life with us. When this co-creation arises unconsciously out of our reactivity, our woundedness, our unexamined habits, greed, aversion, and delusion, then we fall victim to patterns that we are blind to that eat away at the core of our well-being. When we are lucky enough to awaken to our habitual patterns, to see with loving eyes the complex shapes that naturally arise when our vulnerabilities interact, then we can consciously, mindfully, join together in co-creating something beautiful, heartfelt, vibrant, and truly intimate. This conscious, artful, courageous, lovingly mindful shared act of creation cannot help but be transformative, calling us to our better angels and truest selves, so that we might do our part to transform the world and save all beings.

Mindful Mantra

When friction or conflict arises between us, I vow to pay close attention to my own habitual ways of reacting in both body and mind.

May I wake up to my part in the relationship patterns that create distance between us and cause us both to suffer.

May my growing awareness of my patterns be a source of healing and intimacy between me and my beloved, for ourselves and for all beings.

May all beings find the courage to turn toward what they have been turning away from.

May we all welcome what we have made unwelcome.

May we continuously awaken to the compassion and wisdom that are our birthright and our salvation.

May we together co-create an ever-unfolding moment of true intimacy, unity, connection, and love.

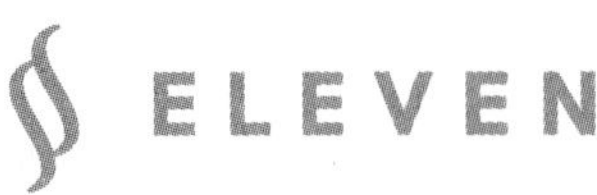

Encountering the Arising of Conflict

ONLY BY LOVE ALONE

Conflict is a naturally arising, inevitable, and perennial element of life. It is normal and healthy and an essential gateway to liberation. Within any relationship, but particularly within one in which we have stepped forward into our vulnerability, we will regularly step on each other's toes, find ourselves at cross-purposes, discover competing needs, have differences of opinion, different tastes, different cadences and rhythms, and/or simply be momentarily out of sync. What we have discovered within relationship science is that it isn't the presence or absence of conflict that makes or breaks a relationship; it is how we encounter conflict, how we behave when in conflict, how carefully we communicate, and how skillfully we repair that makes all the difference.

It isn't the presence or absence of conflict that makes or breaks a relationship; it is how we encounter conflict, how we behave when in conflict, how carefully we communicate, and how skillfully we repair that makes all the difference.

In the spiritual practice of intimacy, it is within the crucible of conflict that we are given the opportunity to encounter ourselves at our most reactive and raw. It is within conflict that our ego asserts itself most ferociously and becomes both most solid and fragile. It is within conflict that our vulnerabilities are most threatened and thus where our most destructive habits of self-protection and defensiveness are most likely to arise. It is within conflict that we are most likely to turn away from intimacy and connection. And, simultaneously, it is within conflict that we are repeatedly granted the opportunity to practice the kind of turning toward and opening up that ultimately erodes the barriers that separate us from each other and from our true selves.

Conflict Within: Practicing Intimacy with the Roots of Conflict

Conflict in our relationship begins with conflict within ourselves. Within each of us is a lifetime of accumulated wounds, established vulnerabilities, and inherited destructive habits that we bring with us into our relationships. As we turn to examine deeply the roots of conflict in our own being, we begin to free ourselves and our partners from these ancient streams of suffering, so that we might experience more love and joy and so that our children might be spared this awful inheritance.

Often our conflictual reactivity is rooted in our vulnerability. Instinctively we ferociously protect our vulnerability. The protection can take the form of either hiddenness or lashing out. We lash out to protect our vulnerability, but at some level we are also ashamed of our vulnerability. You may recall from Chapter 2 that we hate our vulnerability and wish we could cut it out and throw it away. We carry our vulnerability as a curse. We hold our vulnerability at arm's length, as something vile that must be discarded or as a problem that must be solved. We turn away from and judge our own vulnerability, and when others get close to it or threaten it, we fight. This is the deepest root of conflict.

As we try to solve the problem of our vulnerability primarily by hiding it and hiding from it, we make ourselves strangers to the world and to ourselves. We don't let others really know us, and we don't really know or accept ourselves. When we are hurt, we hurt others. When we are hurt, we defend ourselves and criticize others. We snarl and snap, or whimper and moan. We blame and call names. We make others wrong to try to make ourselves right. We vilify and condemn. We go to war. And that war may be either hot or cold, but either way it cleaves the world into "us" and "them" and commits the great sin of separation.

Conflict Between: It Takes Two to Tug-of-War

In all conflict, as we say, it takes two to tango. Conflict emerges when there is separation, and we take up arms on our side against the other. It's as though, as soon as someone takes up one end of the tug-of-war rope, we are immediately pulled into the nightmare of separation, with the rope melded to our hands. Then, when they pull, we must pull back. They pull south, and we pull north. However, if someone picks up the rope, and we do not pick up the other side, then there is only one person dragging a rope around. No conflict. No war. Just a slack rope.

What welds our hands to the other side of the rope?

Attachment. Attachment to our ego. Attachment to our mission to hide and protect our vulnerability at any cost. For instance, if we see ourself as generous but our partner calls us cheap, we must go to war to protect our view of ourself as generous. If we want to be seen as harmless, but our partner says we caused them harm, we go to war to defend our view of ourself as harmless. If we feel tired and overburdened, and our partner asks us to do the dishes, we go to war to protect our exhaustion. We will go to war to assert our desire to be cared for. We will go to war to protect our view of ourself as admirable and gentle. We will go to war to protect others who matter to us.

What welds our hands to the rope is our own unexamined karma—the ways in which our experience has taught us that going to war is the only option. And it is the fact that we are welded to the rope that steals our freedom and makes us and all others captive to our reactivity. If we are welded to the rope, and we think our partner *might* pick up the other end, then we must start pulling, whether we really want to or not. And if we start pulling and our beloved's hand is also welded to the rope, then we are both trapped, each feeling we must pull with all our might until someone wins, is exhausted, or dies.

So, when we look deeply at the roots of conflict in our relationships, we see that our vulnerabilities are the rope, that perceived threats to our vulnerability are the other end of the rope, that our conviction that our vulnerability must be defended at all costs is what welds us to the rope, and that our reactive defensiveness is our enslavement to pulling.

Miscommunication

Perhaps more often than not, when we stumble into each other's vulnerabilities and cause hurt and harm, it is through simple miscommunication and misinterpretation. Miscommunication is the rule, not the exception. We say something that to us means, "Isn't this a funny call back to a show that we watched together?" and our partner hears, "Remember that horribly shameful thing you did three years ago?" And the next thing you know, we're arguing about something that to us seems like a complete non sequitur and that to our partner seems like a deliberate assault.

Why is miscommunication more the norm than the exception in our relationships? Because we each have a different personal history, and even though on the surface it may appear that we are speaking exactly the same language and living in exactly the same reality, in practice even simple words or experiences can have at least subtle if not vastly different meanings to each of us. For example, to me *intimacy* means the lived experience of our deepest interconnectedness. To others, *intimacy* means sex. Whenever I start talking about intimacy with a new couple, I often have to clarify what I mean quickly; otherwise, they assume I'm only talking about sex, rather than talking more broadly about interconnection and vulnerability that is inclusive of but not limited to sex.

Another example, less about the meaning of words and more about the meaning of experiences, might be that, to me, gentle teasing is a way to express affection and acceptance, and to others teasing is primarily experienced as criticizing and rejecting. So I might be trying to communicate closeness, and my partner might hear rejection. Miscommunication at its finest.

Between two partners, each is speaking a dialect of a similar language built out of each of their own accumulated histories of personal experiences and meaning making. To Aiyanna, spending more time together elicits images of snuggling on the couch and long lunches over tea. To Miguel, spending more time together elicits images of hiking through the mountains, going kayaking together, and making love. You can see how conflict can arise in a seemingly mystifying way as each tries to move toward what they thought was a shared vision of spending more time together, only to end up feeling frustrated and rejected. He's loading the kayaks and she's thinking, "Why doesn't he want to snuggle with me?" She's inviting him to hang out on the couch, and he's thinking, "Why doesn't she ever want to do anything with me?"

Grist for the Mill

Skillful action during conflict begins with mindfulness of our inner experience, so that we might hold ourselves with compassion and transform what is happening between us into wisdom. In both therapy and contemplative practice, we often say that everything is grist for the mill. The phrase *grist for the mill* brings to mind something that is coarse and rough being offered to the millstone to be transformed into something fine and smooth. This practice of being awake and cultivating intimacy in the middle of conflict epitomizes this saying in that what we are experiencing in our bodies and minds feels so coarse and rough that it pushes us to act coarsely and roughly. Encountering and embracing it feels abrasive and painful. And yet, when we give it all to the millstone of our mindfully intimate practice, we can transform it into something fine and good, something that connects us and makes us wiser, better, and more useful.

> Aiyanna and Miguel were on the second-to-last day of their vacation, and Aiyanna asked Miguel what he wanted to do before they returned home. Miguel responded by expressing his hope to get a chance to finish writing the proposal he had been working on for months. She got quiet for several minutes. After waiting a while to see if she would start to open up again, he asked, "Did I say something that hurt your feelings?"
>
> Aiyanna paused for a long time, took a deep breath, and said, "I asked about fun and joyful experiences that we could have together, and you responded about work. It feels like we aren't on the same page and like you aren't even listening to me."
>
> Miguel felt criticized and reacted, "Are you kidding me? You asked what I wanted to do, and now you're mad at me because I didn't give you the answer you wanted? I just answered honestly. I didn't know I was supposed to read your mind."
>
> Aiyanna reacted by saying, "Fine, if you'd rather work than spend time with me, then just take me home."
>
> Both could feel the coarse and rough grist for the mill churning through their bodies. Miguel had answered his wife's question honestly,

and he had a powerful urge to defend it. His reactivity in that moment was rooted in his own vulnerability to feeling that other people don't really care to hear about his authentic experience. Aiyanna, on the other hand, is vulnerable to feeling that time has been squandered rather than spent savoring connection. So, when she is imagining a moment where she thought they might go hiking together but instead finds him deeply absorbed in typing, she feels lonely and hurt.

When stung, Aiyanna tends to withdraw, and Miguel tends to poke and prod. They both worked to be heard. They both defended themselves. They struggled. It hurt. The grist was still coarse and rough.

So where are the keys to liberation?

Setting the Intention to Awaken to Hurt

Here, at the root of conflict, we find gate after gate that we can unlock with the keys of an ever-deepening intimacy with ourselves and each other. So we set our intention to try to wake up during moments of conflict so that we might practice turning toward the intensity of our experience with love and courage.

When our beloved tells us that we have hurt or angered them because it seems like we don't care, we will immediately feel hurt and defensive. This is an event primed for conflict. But we can remember the vow to take up the practice of turning toward intimacy. Right here, in the heart of the emotional maelstrom we are experiencing, is where we can find our intention to wake up, to pause and take some time to feel deeply into our reaction with loving curiosity. To realize that this moment of conflict is a golden opportunity for us to live up to our intention to practice faithful and determined attention.

Paying Attention to Conflict

The practice of intimacy through conflict involves turning toward these moments of conflict arising from miscommunication with curiosity and allowing the mystery of not knowing what is really going on. So how does one actually engage this practice of attention? Here are three steps.

AWAKENING OUR AWARENESS

1. **Find your cushion.** Take any upset you might be feeling arising from conflict, or even the thought or memory of conflict, to the cushion of your regular meditation practice. When you sit down on your cushion or chair, upright and still, you are in the perfect posture to simply receive with steadiness all the tumult that is arising in your heart and mind. Observe thoughts of persecution, judgment, criticism, and defense and greet them with awareness and kindness. You might say to yourself, "Yep, these are exactly the thoughts that always arise when I am upset like this." Notice that these thoughts are neither true nor untrue. Noticing them with mindfulness places them and us in our proper places.

   Also meet your arising emotions. Anger. Sadness. Shame. Fear. Hurt. Worry. Pain. Also Love. Longing. Missing. Need. Desire. Confusion. When you gently acknowledge the presence of strong or subtle emotions, you might notice that you are already hosting them perfectly well, without harm to yourself or anyone else. It is only in reacting against their presence that you create harm.

2. **Find your body.** Ask yourself, "Where are my anger, sadness, and hurt located physically?" Explore those sensations minutely to directly experience all the variety, granularity, and nuance in their moment-to-moment arising. Discover that your emotional experience is essentially ephemeral. Over time spent sitting in awareness, the arising of bodily sensations that you identify as hurt— sad, angry, frustrated, irritated, and so forth—are not at all as solid and heavy as first experienced. When felt directly and deeply, they are constantly changing, flowing, becoming, arising, and passing away, with nothing coherent or solid at the center.

   It is this flow that you are invited to rest in. Let your body float along inside the moving current of arising experience, without effort or resistance. It is here precisely where you can encounter a resilience born of connection with all things. You are perfectly capable of hosting even the strongest emotional experiences with intimacy and grace. When you have encountered this aspect of your most fundamental nature, then you become capable of true intimacy with yourself, with each other, and with the entire universe.

3. **Name the grist.** Conflict arises for so many reasons: miscommunication, different wants and needs, different opinions, and simply different ways of being in the world. You stumble into each other's vulnerable spots and trigger reactivities. So the practice is to let go of your certainty that you are perceiving things accurately and your certainty that your partner

is misperceiving things. Acknowledge that two different truths can be simultaneously present and that you may only be partially aware of either of them.

When you can humbly start from the presumption that miscommunication is more common than not, you can practice bringing to bear your willingness to be curious and to learn from your partner and from yourself the difference between what was said and what was heard, the difference between what was meant and what was received.

Skillful Action: Practicing Intimacy in the Midst of Conflict

I often note that it is possible to wake up at any point before, during, or after conflict, but in lived experience there is often a developmental sequence to this growing capacity for mindful awareness.

Waking up after conflict. Most often we begin by waking up *after* a conflict has already played itself totally out, and our physiology has begun to return to baseline. We "come back to our senses." The intensity of our emotional experience has ebbed away, and we are able, if we are able, to let go of our commitment to fight or flight and maybe to seek to repair the connection that has been broken.

Waking up before conflict. With more practice, on and off the cushion, we will become more and more available to wake up *before* conflict arises, noticing ourselves on the edge of digging in our spurs and galloping full throttle into war, and therefore able to hold back the reins, breathe deeply, return to our mindful presence with mind and body, and continue to take good care of ourselves, our partner, and our open connection. Waking up before conflict gets emotionally heated is somewhat easier exactly because we are not yet drowning in stress "fight-or-flight" hormones and still have access to the executive function areas of our frontal lobes.

Waking up during conflict. However, when we are flooded with stress hormones, when conflict has arisen strongly in our bodies and minds, and between us and our partner, then waking up to mindful presence can be especially difficult to conjure. Thus the most difficult time to wake up and stay mindful is *during* conflict. However, it is precisely during conflict that perhaps the most fruitful intimacy practice can occur.

Right during conflict, if we are awake to it, we can notice the arising of all the familiar tensions in the body and all the familiar thoughts in the mind. We can notice the arising of impulses to behave reactively—for example, to start raising our voice. Or we might notice the arising of the impulse to withdraw and get sullenly quiet. We might imagine getting up and storming off or driving away. We might catch ourselves right on the cusp of saying something critical or defensive or mean. Right here, embroiled in the stew of strong emotions and unhelpful thoughts, we can practice the attunement of stop, drop, and roll (see Chapter 9), bringing our mindful attention to hold gently the powerful sensations in the body and the overly certain thoughts of the mind.

Right in the midst of feeling misunderstood, we can warmly acknowledge our own pain *and* seek instead to understand our partner's. Right in the middle of feeling hurt, we can hold our hurt close to our heart *and* seek to see, touch, acknowledge, and soothe our partner's hurt. Right amid wanting desperately to run away, we can warmly hold our wish to escape *and* stay present and engaged with our partner—only seeking to be understood *after* we have sought to compassionately understand.

Right in the middle of feeling hurt, we can hold our hurt close to our heart *and* seek to see, touch, acknowledge, and soothe our partner's hurt.

We can simply notice all the powerful forces that are arising and choose to refrain from enacting them. If we can do that one simple thing, that thing that we practice over and over again on the meditation cushion—present-centered stillness—then we become embodiments of non-harm.

When we can practice being spaciously mindful of all our inner turmoil during a moment of conflict between us and our partners, then we can practice true intimate relating. We can practice mindful and gentle speech. We can practice careful and gentle bodily presence. We can practice empathy and clear communication that creates connection and understanding, rather than separation and harm.

We can also practice repair, which is absolutely essential if we want to create and maintain healthy, happy, vibrant intimate relationships. We cover forgiveness at length in the next chapter.

Reaching through the Dragon

The practice of reaching through the dragon is the practice of seeing through our partner's anger to touch their pain. Anger and other hard emotional expressions are always rooted in pain and vulnerability. And yet, even though our partner is in pain, when they express that pain through anger, all we make contact with is anger. When they express that pain as withdrawal, all we make contact with is withdrawal. Relationship scientists have shown us that anger and withdrawal are like magnets in interpersonal interaction. Anger attracts anger. It is also why conflict tends to escalate so quickly and toward such boringly predictable conclusions. We are on automatic pilot, simply reacting and reacting without mindfulness and care.

Reaching through the dragon requires that we be awake to our own reactivity in a moment of conflict so that we can hold our reactivity with care and awareness. We hold our reactivity with care and awareness so that we might, rather than reacting to anger with anger, reach through our partner's anger to touch their pain, respond with compassion, care, and understanding.

For example, if our partner is angry with us because we're not taking their concerns seriously, we can notice our own anger and defensiveness arising, and rather than falling into fight or flight, we can see that they're in pain and maybe say, "I'm sorry. It feels awful to feel like I'm not taking you seriously. Please let me try again. Tell me a little bit more about what's worrying you." In this way, we are addressing the source of our partner's pain nondefensively, rather than simply perpetuating conflict by meeting anger with anger. This is skillful means. This is the practice of serving the connecting experience of intimacy rather than the separating experience of conflict.

Often, when we are able to reach through the dragon to touch our partner's pain, their anger diffuses, and we're able to connect and work together toward deepening understanding.

The spiritual practice involves experiencing both our own reactivity and our partner's reactivity with compassion, without separation, and without having to defend our ego. It means being able to serve a higher ideal than simply giving in to fight or flight.

MINDFUL ATTUNEMENT TO CONFLICT

As you practice, consider saying these things to yourself as they apply:

- It is the ego that separates me from my partner and from all other beings. It even separates me from myself.
- When I take up the practice of intimacy in the midst of conflict, it is possible to see through the illusion that my ego is solid and must be defended at all costs.
- When I take up the practice of intimacy, I begin to cultivate a capacity to see through my ego and my partner's ego, so that I can know that we are not separate and that my pain is their pain and their pain is mine.
- It is possible to learn not just to become more skillful in our relationships but to truly wake up to the wholeness that has always been our birthright.

As you practice, consider saying these things to your partner as they apply:

- My dear one, I can see that your pain and mine are not separate.
- I know in my bones that tending to your pain is also tending to my own.
- When I hurt you, I hurt myself. When I indulge in anger and conflict, I cannot help but cause harm to all that I love.
- I vow to meet moments of conflict with compassion and wisdom, so that I and you and the world together might wake up to our true nature.

Miguel and Aiyanna struggled for longer than either of them wanted to. They both felt exhausted and a bit sad. Milling the grist for Miguel meant engaging his practice of stop, drop, and roll. Right there, he took a long deep breath and let himself become still and quiet. He stopped adding fuel to the fire. He turned his attention to the distress he was feeling in his body—feeling it, breathing into it, and allowing himself to be intimate with it. It felt terrible, and he stayed with it like a parent rocking an upset child.

Then he turned his attention to the thoughts arising in his mind. Thoughts of storming off. Thoughts of saying defensive and offensive things. He noticed how common those thoughts are when he's upset and felt how common they must be for everyone under similar circumstances. He felt some compassion for himself, his body, and his mind.

This wasn't a straightforward, linear experience. It involved several trial-and-error attempts to work with his own reactive body and mind, while reminding himself of his commitment to finding a more relationally skillful way forward.

He asked himself, "What can I do now that will actually be skillful, that will help us repair and reconnect?" That question helped him remember that empathizing with Aiyanna's pain rather than defending his own always works better in the service of intimacy. He wanted to reach through the dragon of anger and connect with her hurt. Putting himself in Aiyanna's shoes, he imagined that Aiyanna was experiencing quite a bit of sadness about their vacation coming to an end. She felt pressure to make sure they made the most of their time together before returning to the seemingly constant grind of their everyday work lives. She was hoping to play and daydream and seize the last few moments of nonresponsible adult life.

Miguel also acknowledged that he was feeling a strong call to finish his proposal while his attention wasn't being grabbed by a million different demands. He realized that they were both seeking more ease, rest, and connection. They just had different visions of the path and sequence of steps to that end.

Finally, he turned toward Aiyanna and shared that his initial response to her question had been hurtful and that he had only added to that hurt with his defensiveness. He apologized for hurting her and for being reactive. He shared with her his growing understanding of why what he said hurt her, because she yearned to connect in the time they had left, and he had responded by saying he wanted to do solo activities like exercise and writing. Then he added insult to injury by becoming reactively defensive. He took responsibility for his unskillful defensiveness and vowed to try to do better in the future.

For her part, Aiyanna expressed her care for Miguel's sadness about vacation ending and his anxiety about making more progress on the proposal while there was still time. She apologized for reacting, withdrawing, and leading with anger and vowed to try to move more quickly toward sharing the hurt without blame, helping them both move back toward being in sync when misunderstandings naturally arise.

When Miguel and Aiyanna were able to see and touch each other's pain and worry, acknowledge that they understood where the other was coming from, and genuinely and compassionately communicate their care for each other, the conflict just. . . . dissipated. The residue of reactive conflict can continue to ache for a little while, but the balm of repair and reconnection always heals.

Unsolvable Problems

Some problems just don't lend themselves to easy solutions. In fact, some of the sources of greatest conflict in our relationships are, for all practical purposes, unsolvable. It is, however, not the fact that they are unsolvable that destroys our intimate connection but, instead, the fact that we continue to struggle with them as though they could be solved. We struggle as though, with just a little more effort, insistence, or anger, resolution will happen. Or we withdraw, accumulating resentment, because we are convinced that the problem would be solved if only our partner would stop being so stubborn or selfish. We fail to fully recognize these friction points in our relationships as unsolvable by their nature and to therefore consider the possibility that their unsolvability may be a gift. In other words, what if the unsolvability of this problem is a feature and not a bug?

If we are to take intimacy as a spiritual practice seriously, then our unsolvable problems become some of our most generous and effective teachers. Few things play as roughly with the ego as unsolvable problems, both in general and more specifically in our relationships. The ego wants what it wants when it wants it: "I want a solution to my problem so that I can feel better now." Of course we want that. And it is not necessarily a bad thing to want. When a problem is genuinely solvable, and the solution does more good than harm, then actively solving our problems is exactly the most generous and healthy thing to do. But when the problem does not lend itself to a solution, or the solution does more harm than good, then continuing to struggle with it is just like beating your head against the wall—painful and pointless.

Consider, for example, one couple I worked with in which one of the most significant sources of conflict and distress arose from the fact that one partner was more naturally drawn to polyamory as a way of being in relationship, and the other partner was more naturally drawn to monogamy. In this relationship, one partner cannot live their preference without great cost to the other partner. They cannot be both actively polyamorous and strictly monogamous. There is no middle ground. They can't just take turns living their preference without greatly constricting and hurting one another. And, for this couple, they do not consider splitting up a solution that would be worth the cost. If, however, we begin to consider this difference as simply a difference, if we choose to honor that both partners have a right to want what they want, and if we grant that one way of being is not necessarily right and the other necessarily wrong, *then* what becomes most vividly apparent?

In other words, if we practice allowing ourselves to be intimate with everything that is simultaneously true and allow our body, mind, and heart to be a large and spacious container within which all contradictions can be held with gentleness and care, then we begin to embody a life of grace, humility, and peace. Living the contradictions, the contrasts, the unsolvabilities with integrity and clarity is the intimate path.

Is there an unsolvable problem in your relationship? It may be something small and minor in the grand scheme of your relationship, or it may be a regular source of significant painful conflict. Whatever it is, it will surely be characterized by a feeling that there is no resolution that fully satisfies both of you. If one of you "wins," the other "loses." If you settle on an answer to the problem, no matter what it is, the answer is somehow just wrong. Whether it is going out or staying in (something relatively small) or practicing monogamy or consensual nonmonogamy (something relatively big), there is no ideal solution that makes both partners happy.

So how do we practice intimacy together with an unsolvable problem?

Moving Forward with the Unsolvable Problem

In searching for an answer to how we might practice intimacy in the face of an unsolvable problem, we can find a clue, albeit a mysterious one, in a famous koan, a traditional means of intimacy practice in Zen. In this particular koan story, a teacher named Yen Kuan was feeling the heat of the day and called out to his attendant in the other room, "Please bring me the rhinoceros fan." The rhinoceros horn fan was a gift that the teacher had been given by the emperor. The attendant, however, came in and said, "I'm so sorry. The fan is broken." Yen Kuan looked up at him and said, "Then bring me the rhinoceros." The attendant just stood in the doorway and didn't know what to say or what to do.

And that's it. That is the heart of the koan. It gently guides us into a moment in which we can bring neither the fan nor the rhinoceros. We are stuck. The problem has no solution. So what do we do? Just as we do in our relationship when we can neither go through nor around some issue between us. We cannot be both monogamous and polyamorous. We cannot both go out and stay in. We cannot raise our children both secular and religious.

In the koan, a teacher, years later, responds to the story of the rhinoceros fan by simply drawing a circle and writing the word *rhinoceros* in it. In my mind, I imagine the joy and laughter of the group as they meet this playful way forward.

So, in our relationships, we just move forward.

Intention, Attention, and Action with an Unsolvable Problem

The first step is to simply stop struggling to solve the unsolvable. This step can be difficult, especially if we have already invested a lot of time and effort in trying to solve the problem. It can be hard to arrest the momentum of problem-solving efforts that we have generated because it feels so much like giving up and too close to hopeless resignation. But, if we remind ourselves that we can always pick the struggle back up again if we absolutely have to and that we'll only be practicing putting it down for a little while, that might be just reassuring enough to allow us to relax and let it go for just a moment.

When we are in sitting meditation, we can notice that we are feeling the desperation for a solution arising in our body. We notice the arising of wanting to have things our way and how desperate we can be to win. We notice the arising of the hopelessness that follows feeling frustrated by our failure to struggle our way to a solution. We notice how we compulsively pick up the problem again and again, each time hoping anew that this time we will find the solution that has eluded us for so long. We notice how this unquenchable wanting compels so much of our attention and narrows our focus to a pinpoint on just this problem and its lack of solution. We can feel for the flow and nuance of those sensations with a gentle curiosity that allows us to simply notice it without becoming fused to it—to feel it without falling for it. We can say to ourselves, "Ah, this is what yearning for a solution feels like. I can sit with this. I can breathe with this. For these few moments I can just want a solution in the absence of having a solution. I can experience this without harm."

And right here in the middle of a sea of wanting and not having, we might begin to notice that we are already living quite well and quite vividly in a world with no solutions. Sipping our coffee. Walking our dog. Doing our work. Washing the dishes. The world with no solutions in it is in actuality quite wide and full of wonders too vast and subtle to ever tire of. In the midst of our dissatisfaction with having no answer to our problem, we simultaneously swim in a sea of satisfaction with the richness of our unfathomable lives. Let us notice this. Let the breath hold us. Let our coffee cup and the blue sky welcome us. We make our bed. Pay our bills. Let our life unfold. Savor this solution-free world.

When there is no perfect solution, we move forward with just what we have in our pockets and in our hearts and the blessing of no unassailably right answer, no ultimate resolution. In Zen practice, we sometimes note the great freedom that arises from recognizing that all answers are provisional and imperfect. We are invited to live joyously into the dynamic truth that is this ceaselessly unfolding moment of one continuous mistake.

Knowing and caring in this dynamic space is the key to preserving and practicing intimacy. We say something like, "I know that our current 'solution' is imperfect, and I care about what it costs you—you care about what it costs me. We do not dismiss each other or turn away from what we are creating together. We live this moment fully for all its richness, in the absence of a solution. Reveling in not knowing."

Some couples, for example, choose monogamy and forgo polyamory, knowing and caring that this choice has costs and benefits, both known and unknown, for both partners. And they live into it. They go to movies together, they make love, they make dinner, they argue about nothing in particular, they make up, they snuggle, and they set the alarm for six.

Other couples choose consensual nonmonogamy and forgo monogamy, knowing and caring that this choice has costs and benefits, both known and unknown for both partners. And they live into it. They plant gardens and raise rabbits. They cut firewood and go grocery shopping. They argue about money and hold hands while waiting in line. They talk to friends, and file taxes, and laugh at jokes no one else on earth understands.

They draw circles and write the word *rhinoceros* in them.
And laugh.

The Heart of the Matter

Points of friction are a natural part of interacting with any other human being. Our wants and needs will sometimes be at odds. We will trigger our partner, and our partner will trigger us. We bring our vulnerabilities and unexamined reactivities into all our relationships. We suffer from conflict. And yet, on the path of intimacy, moments of conflict are some of our most important teachers. We are given opportunities, through conflict, again and again to wake up to our habits of body and mind that harden our ego and separate us from each other. As we warmly meet our partner's armored tenderness, we learn to see clearly and act with compassion and wisdom, such that they might also experience less separation and more intimacy.

We must also acknowledge that life and love are full of puzzles with no solutions. As with all suffering, our agony arises from our desperate desire to make reality and our relationship bend to our wishes. And yet freedom and joy are available and waiting for us right here in a world without answers. The sun rises and sets. Precious beings are born and die. Spring blossoms smell like happiness, and winter chills our bones. This contradictory, unsolvable love is right here in our hands to be savored. Savor it together.

Mindful Mantra

My dearest one, I vow with you and with all beings
To wake up to my ancient reactivities
And to reach through your armor to touch your true heart.
I vow not to allow conflict to obscure our hearts' connection.
I vow not to turn away, but only toward.
May you and I and all beings know the peace that arises when all conflict turns to knowing
And when all strife turns to intimacy.
May we love each other completely amid the folly of our lives.
May we practice lovingly with problems that cannot be solved.

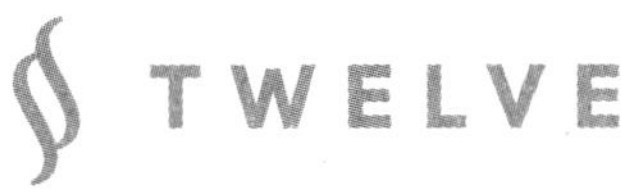

TWELVE

Repairing Ruptures

TO MEND WHAT HAS BEEN BROKEN

Because you are, and I am, and everyone else is, vulnerable, we will all experience hurt. In my relationship, my partner will cause me some measure of pain virtually every day, and I in turn will cause my partner some measure of pain every day. Not necessarily on purpose. Not out of vindictiveness or malevolence. More often than not, simply out of ignorance, misunderstanding, or thoughtlessness. Right there, in an ocean of love and care, sweetness, sensuality, and compassion, there will be pain. And how we come to terms with that pain, how we meet it and respond to it, makes all the difference in whether we continue to nurture and grow our intimate connection or let it burn and crumble.

Given that intimate relationship means that we will hurt our partner through what we do and fail to do, through what we say and fail to say, and that we will experience feeling hurt by our partner through what they do and fail to do, through what they say and fail to say, this chapter is about how we can walk the path of *repair, atonement,* and *forgiveness*—again and again, over and over, for the rest of our short, sweet lives.

Repair

Learning how to repair things is an essential life skill. Nowhere is this more important than in our intimate relationships. Repair is a skill that we bring to the smaller day-to-day hurts and stings that are part and parcel of a life lived in close emotional and physical proximity. We do our best to continually practice mindfulness in our relationships, treating our partner with gentleness, care, kindness, compassion, tenderness, love, respect, and joy. However, it is simply our human nature to be at times also thoughtless, gruff, irritable, frustrated, cranky, inattentive, short, harsh, argumentative, defensive, angry, demanding, critical, and complaining. All this fussiness, though inescapably human, causes harm nonetheless. This fact can be hard for us to accept.

The vast majority of couples that I know and work with not only consistently fail to notice and repair these day-to-day hurts in their relationships, but they actually feel irritated by the notion that they should have to be careful of and seek to repair the small thoughtless hurts that they cause throughout the day: "I don't want to have to go around apologizing for every little thing all day long. My partner should just grow a thicker skin and let it roll off their back."

And this is the casually mundane way that we all turn away from intimacy. We turn away from the little day-to-day hurts because they just feel too frequent and too hard to keep up with. We get frustrated and irritated at how often we hurt our partner's feelings. Or we get fed up with how often our partner hurts our feelings. And we turn away.

The Porcupines' Dilemma

In Arthur Schopenhauer's Porcupines' Dilemma, one cold day a group of porcupines seeking the comfort of each others' warmth began to huddle together, snuggling close and savoring the loveliness of heat and connection. "This is cozy," they all thought, "but these damn quills keep poking me!" No matter how they each tried, they couldn't avoid being poked at least a little bit by the others' quills. So they all pulled away from each other, treasuring the relief of no longer being pricked and poked. However, soon enough they were all freezing again, so once again sought to snuggle together for comfort and warmth. And, once again, they started poking each other. Caught between these two discomforts, what do the poor porcupines do?

What do we, poor porcupines, do?

I think for most of us, we resolve our own personal porcupines' dilemma by pulling back just far enough to avoid each other's quills and simply giving up on the warmth of getting any closer. For most couples, the solution is "as close as we can tolerate, but no closer." And so, like the porcupines, we are, as a result, always at least a little bit cold, always at least a little bit lonely, isolated, and separate.

Maybe if our partner is a little irritable or withdrawn, we learn to cope by doing our best not to care. If our partner is predictably critical or complaining, maybe we withdraw, hide, or try to learn not to care, to not let it bother us. And when we do this, eventually we really don't care, and it really doesn't bother us. Now the distance between us has frozen, and we just get used to being cold, thinking this is normal, this is what being in a relationship is like, and so we just get on with the business of getting through our days.

In relation to our own quills, maybe at first we try our best to keep them down and to move carefully and cautiously to minimize how often we stick our partner. Maybe when we do stick our partner, we apologize and adjust a little bit to try to stop poking them or at least to minimize the pain we are causing. But, eventually, it's just a lot of effort and involves too much contorting, so we relax and let our quills hang however they want.

In this place, maybe we tell our partner to stop being so sensitive and to stop blaming us for every little time we accidentally poke them. We may say something like, "You know I don't mean anything by it. Just let it go." So, again, we try to learn not to care when we poke our partner. Or maybe, because we can't avoid it and they are just going to go around being hurt by us anyway, we start poking them on purpose out of irritation and spite. Maybe when they poke us, we poke them back harder to "show them how it feels." We learn to harden our heart to our partner's pain. And, when we do this, something inside us freezes, and now we don't have to try anymore; we honestly just don't care about our partner's pain anymore. We start to think that this is normal. This is just how relationships are. We get used to being cold and to seeing our partner being cold. We turn instead to the busyness of our day and our life.

Although this is how most of us resolve the porcupines' dilemma, this is not the practice of true intimacy. In the practice of true intimacy, we do not settle for separation as the solution to life's pain. In the practice of intimacy, we commit ourselves to connection, to wholeness, to turning toward one another.

Intention, Attention, and Action with Repair

As always, the answer begins with setting our intention. We set our intention to notice and not turn away from the little day-to-day hurts—both the ones we cause and the ones we suffer. We set our intention to notice moments of hurt with clarity and compassion, to turn toward these hurts with gentleness and care. We set our intention to actively repair the hurts we cause and to actively seek repair and offer forgiveness for the hurts we receive. We set our intention to practice the intimacy of repair again and again, every time, forever. We set the intention to take up this spiritual practice for our awakening and for the benefit of all beings.

Next is mindful attention to our quills and attention, care, and repair for the harms we cause. When we poke our partner, we must acknowledge that we've done so and do what we reasonably can to stop actively poking. We can turn toward the little drop of blood arising from the place we poked and tend to it with loving care. We can say, "Oh, I'm so sorry, my love. Let me take care of that." We must do this every time, or as close to every time as we can. That may mean that we're always in some way adjusting, poking, tending, learning, and moving. Each time, we learn a little something more about how to be close to our partner without poking too much.

This capacity to pay attention, notice, and turn toward with loving care is what we are cultivating in our ongoing meditation practice. We practice to learn how to allow ourselves to be poked—allowing and accepting that, if we're going to snuggle in here with our heart wide open and receive the warmth and love and joy that is available to us, then getting poked a little bit from time to time is just the price of admission. So we do our best to accept it with grace and gratitude, authentically experiencing the pokes we receive without blame, resentment, or malice. We can remind ourselves, "My experience of hurt is *my* experience of hurt. It exists wholly within my body and mind, and it is therefore mine to care for with love and wisdom. My hurt is my gateway into mindful intimacy practice."

If we make this moment of hurt about our partner, then we lose the opportunity to practice intimacy with our own experience. And it is intimacy with our own experience that releases us from ancient habit patterns, so that we might feel a deeper connection to our partner and begin to practice more relationally skillful responses.

Of course, we can only really stay openhearted if our partner also lovingly shows that they care when they poke us. This is the *both–and* of intimacy practice. In Zen communities, we say that we are 100% responsible for attending lovingly to the pain arising from where our partner poked us *and* we absolutely need our partner's support, empathy, and care.

An additional way of dancing within the porcupines' dilemma involves moving fluidly within the relational space—stepping forward and stepping back—over and over again forever. We step forward into the dynamic space of deep closeness. And then we step back into our independence—to heal, to grow, to play. The key here is that we are not avoiding closeness, and we are not stuck in separateness. We cuddle in close, warmth and quills and all. Then we waddle off to do our separate porcupine things. Then we come together and huddle close again. All with joy. We practice moving freely within the entire space of our lives together—reveling in moments when we are deeply intertwined and equally reveling in moments when we are wholly independent.

Getting poked a little bit from time to time is just the price of admission. So we do our best to accept it with grace and gratitude.

How you and your partner dance together within the porcupines' dilemma will be your own ongoing creative practice, made up of what is most available to each of you given your lifetime experience of being vulnerable. Yet, as long as you are turning toward, you are taking good care of your connection and making intentional progress toward mindful repair.

THE FIVE A'S OF MINDFUL REPAIR

What are the steps to mindful repair?

1. Attend
2. Acknowledge and empathize
3. Apologize
4. Accept responsibility
5. Adapt

Attend: Attending means paying attention to your partner and not turning away from or ignoring times when you sting them. Attending to their pain creates connection, trust, and intimacy. Dismissing their pain as not real or not worthy of care because you didn't mean to hurt them or because they misinterpreted you just adds pain to pain, further breaking connection, corroding trust, and undermining intimacy. It's easy to pretend not to notice when your partner suddenly gets quiet or withdraws or gets defensive or in some other way flinches from being stung. You likely ignore your partner's moment of hurt, hoping that you can just rush past it and get on with the day without having to be derailed by it or made to feel bad for hurting them. You might even be so used to ignoring the little flinches from your partner when you inadvertently sting them that you genuinely stop noticing them altogether. They simply fade into the background and become an invisible part of the distance that has become normal between you. When you notice their pain, breathe, remember your vow of loving care, and turn toward the hurt that you have caused.

Acknowledge and empathize: Whether the pain you caused was entirely inadvertent or arose from a misunderstanding, your partner's pain is real. And because their pain is real, it must be tended to. Openly acknowledge what you have done. Say, "Oh, my love, I stung you." Acknowledging the truth of it is a kind of blessing and the beginning of a balm. It is genuinely feeling the pain you have caused that creates connection and powerful repair. If you aren't making resonant emotional contact with the pain that you've caused, then you are not waking up from the dream of separateness and are a subject operating on an object. You are managing a situation rather than weaving connection. Through empathy, genuinely feel the pain you have caused, and name it.

Apologize: Perhaps gently touch your partner's hand or face, look into their eyes, and say, "Oh, my love, I'm sorry I stung you." Own it. Don't say, "I'm sorry you took it that way"—because that is not a genuine, or helpful, apology. Apologize immediately, without hesitation, and with genuine care. Let yourself genuinely feel their pain and your own, and then express genuine remorse.

Accept responsibility: It is extremely difficult to accept responsibility for even small harms to our partner, primarily because more often than not you have done so unintentionally, and because it is so humbling to admit to yourself that you are so easily capable of thoughtlessly causing harm to the people you love the most. You think, "Because I didn't mean to hurt you, I want to argue that you shouldn't feel hurt." As you learned in Chapter 11, all this does is pile on more hurt. Accepting responsibility communicates to your partner that you care and that you are not careless or dismissive of even the inadvertent harm that you can cause. This helps your partner (and in the reverse direction, yourself) to feel more intimately safe, seen, and cared for. It communicates that you will be more careful in the future and therefore less likely to cause the same harm. Accepting responsibility simply acknowledges your partner's pain in the same way you would accept responsibility for accidently bumping into someone and knocking them down. You'd say, "Oh, I'm so sorry. Here, let me help you up. Are you okay?" You wouldn't say, "Why did you fall down? I didn't mean to bump into you."

Adapt: Adapting means thoughtfully considering how you might avoid causing the same harm in the future. Sometimes this is something easy to achieve, like promising to not bring up politics again at the next family gathering. Sometimes, however, it is more difficult, like not withdrawing when we've been stung. Openly acknowledge that this is a bit of a growth edge for you, and ask for your partner's help and kind patience in this spot as you continue to learn and adapt. The bottom line is to stay committed to attending mindfully and compassionately to the pain that you cause, even when it is one of the unavoidable quills of porcupine love.

And so repair might be best thought of as something we do early and often for the small day-to-day hurts that are part and parcel of an intimate relationship and the porcupines' dilemma. You sting your partner, you notice, care, feel it, apologize, and adjust. Your partner stings you, and you see that they notice, that they care and feel it, you receive their apology, and you trust their commitment to being gentle with you. That is intimacy.

Atonement

The next level up from repair is atonement. Atonement is the work of mending our connection when we have caused more than a small harm—when we have caused a great harm. What makes the practice of atonement different from the daily practice of repair is that it involves attending to a greater degree of harm, a more profound emotional experience of guilt and shame, a much more extended period of continual apology, and a greater commitment to the lengthy and slow process of regrowing trust and stability.

There are certainly many different ways in which great harm can be caused to a relationship; however, I want to highlight two broad categories: infidelity and attachment injuries.

Infidelity

A wide range of studies have shown that somewhere between 25 and 30% of people self-report having been unfaithful to their committed partners. I am using the terms *infidelity* and *unfaithful* purposefully, because they both represent the breaking of another person's faith and trust. We enter our relationships for the most part freely giving each other the gift of our trust. Then we rest in the trust that our partner will be faithful, and we each consciously accept that trust and willingly take up the responsibility for upholding our partner's faith in us.

However, causes and conditions often conspire such that at least 25–30% of us break our partner's trust by being unfaithful. On the one hand, this relational phenomenon of infidelity is so common that it very clearly arises out of some basic aspect of simply being human. On the other hand, within any particular relationship, such a significant trust violation can be devastating and trigger an existential crisis for both partners. For many couples, the trust breach is simply too severe to be recovered from. Infidelity is often found in studies to be the leading cause of separation and divorce, and more than half of married couples will end their relationship following an extramarital affair. For many couples, infidelity is simply one of the final symptoms of a terminally deteriorating relationship. For others, however, it can be a wake-up call or a reckoning that reorients them back toward their relationship with the determination to heal the wound and move forward together. It is in those cases that we are called to take up the practice of atonement.

Attachment Injury

The second category of great harm is what relationship scientist and clinician Susan Johnson refers to as an attachment injury. Attachment injuries are also trust violations, but they arise out of a specific incident in which one partner fails to meet a moment of significantly acute need for the other.

You might think of this a little bit like a failed trust fall. One partner takes the risk of allowing themself to fall backward, expecting the other partner to catch them; but the other partner fails to catch them, and the first partner gets badly scared and hurt. We count on our partner for connection, soothing, and comfort, and vice versa, especially when we are heartbroken, in agony, or feeling extremely vulnerable. If a partner is not there when most needed, these moments can be devastating to a relationship. These are injuries for which just saying, "I'm so sorry" is insufficient to close the gaping wound. The trust violation gets registered in the bones, and the whole body learns that when the chips are down, the other person cannot be counted on. In these cases of existential trust violation, healing only comes through the practice of atonement.

> Anika's pregnancy was complicated by several factors that affected both her own and the baby's health. As she and Noah moved toward the delivery date, she found herself scared and worried about giving birth and how they would manage her and the baby's needs in the days and weeks afterward. She desperately needed and counted on Noah to be there for both of them, and it was fully his intention to do so. However, within a couple of weeks of her due date, Noah went skiing with a friend he hadn't seen in several years, to get in "one last adventure" before turning the page on his life to being a father and caring for his wife and daughter. Anika was desperately worried that he might get hurt skiing and not be able to be there for her when she needed him most. She all but begged him not to go. But Noah reassured her over and over that it would be all right, that she was anxious about nothing, and that he would be there when she needed him. Despite her worries, he went.
>
> And he fell.
>
> And he shattered his femur.
>
> And Anika went into labor the next day.
>
> He wasn't there for the birth. He wasn't there for the emergency care that Anika needed or their daughter Maya's placement in the NICU. And his injury was so severe that he couldn't be much help or comfort for much of the early weeks home. Just when she needed him most, he wasn't there. Years later, Anika still couldn't really forgive him or trust him. Noah could do nothing to fix what he had broken. They tried to just move past it and get on with the business of parenting

and marriage, but simmering anger, disappointment, hurt, shame, and defensiveness poisoned the space between them.

As we came to see the roots of their distress in this moment of powerful attachment injury, it became clear that if they wanted to move forward together, this years-old, poorly scabbed wound would have to debrided and healed. They needed to move through the process of atonement if forgiveness were ever to have a chance.

The Trust Tree

I often use the image of what I call the *trust tree* when I am working with a couple recovering from infidelity, an attachment injury, or any significant trust breach. In the metaphor, trust is like a great big, beautiful apple tree in the backyard of the house you share with your partner. It is already grown and mature and effortlessly produces gorgeous, sweet apples every season. You both enjoy this inherited bounty and maybe even take it a bit for granted. Then one night, for many reasons both obvious and not, drunk and enamored with the sharpness of your axe, you decide the apple tree is in the way of something else you want (maybe more space or another kind of tree) and you chop it down. The axe is sharp, and the tree is yielding, and you have great fun chopping it down.

And when it's done, you stand amidst the consequences of your actions, realizing that this cannot be undone, and you panic. Maybe you immediately regret it and run inside to confess and throw yourself on the mercy of your partner. Maybe you try to hide it and hope your partner doesn't ever notice. But eventually the truth comes out, and your partner is devastated, and the trust tree is just. . . . gone.

Maybe you try to pick up the fallen tree and hope that you can just pretend it didn't happen. Maybe you try to move on and convince yourself that "we didn't need that tree anyway." But the tree and the trust are gone, and you discover that it was essential to what made you happy and secure in your home.

If you want to move forward together in this home, you have to figure out how to grow a new tree. And, just like a new tree, trust must be grown from a seedling and tended with patient and loving care for a long, long time before it will bear any fruit. The process begins with going out into the backyard and bearing witness to what you have done, then planting the new seedling and dedicating yourself to its health and well-being. You will have to come out here every day to water it and protect it and tend to it with diligence and patience. And you will need your partner's help and cooperation. The tree and the trust will not grow without their presence and engagement, and it is up to you to invite them and reassure them and provide them with whatever they need to be able to join you in the backyard with the fallen tree and the new fledgling tree and the long road ahead and the blue sky and birdsong.

This is the practice of atonement. The metaphor guides us to the patience, steadiness, conscientiousness, and reliability that are necessary to the practice of atonement. It also shows us that atonement must be tended to in the presence of the hurt, regret, shame, and guilt that we experience from our having caused great harm. We are called on to carry this bone-deep lesson with as much grace and dignity as we can muster so that our cultivation of healing can be our highest priority.

Intention, Attention, and Action with Seeking Atonement

When we find ourselves in a moment when we are confronted with some great harm that we have caused, our natural human instinct is to defend ourselves. We want to make excuses for our behavior, we want to minimize the harm that was caused, we want the situation to repair itself quickly and thoroughly so we can just move past this shameful moment and return to the way things were before. All these strategies are ways of turning away.

Remember that intimacy can only ever be rescued by turning *toward*. We must turn toward the harm that we have caused. We must acknowledge that trust in us has been shattered. We must openheartedly receive the embarrassment and shame that arises from having violated our own values and the trust of someone we love. We must turn toward and receive all of this without turning away or denying. And we must often do this in the absence of one of the main people we have usually counted on to have our back, the partner we injured.

In order to do this, we must rely on our root meditation practice and perhaps the help and guidance of a skilled therapist. In our practice, we bring our whole self to the cushion. We sit, upright and still, and bring our attention to the breath. Breathing in and breathing out. We let our body and mind sit and just receive all the thoughts and sensations, no matter how powerful, that are arising out of this moment. Maybe we cry. We most certainly ache. But we don't turn away.

We admit to ourselves that we have caused great harm. We don't try to excuse it. We just acknowledge that it is true. We let ourselves feel the pain of the person we have harmed without protecting ourselves from it. We cultivate thorough and complete empathy and compassion. We also suffer the harm that we have caused. We take our time and are gentle and kind with ourselves. This practice is excruciatingly difficult. We sit for as much time and as many times as it takes, until we know that we can carry this pain. We can carry it with tenderness and determination. Then we stand up from the cushion and step onto the relational path.

The practice of atonement also must involve a period of deep reflection as we seek to discover and understand the root causes that contributed to our harmful actions. We must seek things inside us, or perhaps outside us, that we can endeavor to change and grow so that we are less likely to cause the same kind of harm in the future. Maybe we discover a deep well of self-doubt that makes us susceptible to the flirtatious attention of others. Or maybe we discover a kind of selfishness and reluctance to sacrifice in the service of others. Whatever the source, we can turn toward and bathe it in loving attention so that we might transform it into greater gratitude and generosity. Turning toward might involve therapy and the patience and humility necessary to see old destructive patterns and to grow toward newer and healthier intimate patterns.

We approach our partner and ask if it is a good time to talk. If it is, we admit fully to the harm that we have caused without excuse. We own the pain our partner is experiencing and express our great sorrow. And then we invite them to share all their thoughts and feelings with us, vowing to listen, hear, and understand without defense or judgment. You might say, "My love, I have hurt you so badly. I am so sorry. I realize that I have caused great, and maybe irreparable, harm. I am determined to mend what I have broken, however long it takes. I want to be here for you and to regain your trust. I will listen deeply to everything you have to say. I will speak honestly to anything that you ask me. I will care for your wounded heart in whatever way you need. For weeks, for months, for years, for the rest of my life. I will atone for what I have done."

THE STEPS TO ATONEMENT

Because it bears repeating, let me broadly outline the steps of the practice of atonement one more time. The moment you wake up to the fact that you have done something that has caused great harm will be a very difficult moment emotionally. You may feel overwhelmed, despairing, and lost.

1. *Taking refuge.* Take refuge in your sitting practice. Sit still with the undeniability of the harm you have caused and make room for all that is arising. Feel the body take refuge in the posture, and bring your attention to your breathing. Breathe in and out for however long it takes. Let all the thoughts and powerful feelings arise and dissipate, arise and dissipate, over and over again. Even if it is not obvious in the moment, this sitting practice connects you to your basic fundamental resilience.
2. *Admitting harm.* Be open to the growing clarity of the situation and admit the harm you have caused, your culpability, and your desire to learn from what you have done. Atone.
3. *Inviting understanding.* Invite your partner to share their experience so you can understand the impact even more thoroughly. Practice deep listening (see Chapter 5) without excuse or defense. On the long road of atonement, this practice may be something that you do many times over the weeks and months, giving your partner many opportunities to help you understand their evolving pain.
4. *Doing the individual work.* Do your own individual work to uncover the things about yourself that predisposed you to the actions that caused the harm. Consider how you can grow toward greater trustworthiness. Some of this individual work happens in your meditation practice, and some of it may happen in individual therapy. Embody the practice daily by being relentlessly trustworthy and reliable and by doing better, step after step, for a long, long time.
5. *Doing the couple work.* Together with your partner, actively engage in the relationship work of finding and learning about all the weak spots in yourselves and your relationship that put your relationship at risk. Endeavor to address and strengthen them all. This relationship work almost certainly benefits from the guidance of a skilled couple therapist.

The Humble Intimacy Warrior

What makes all this a spiritual practice is the excruciating practice of humility involved at every step. We experience and learn the stickiness of our own ego, the places where our ego made excuses for our actions, and the ways in which our ego will rise up again and again to defend itself from the consequences. The practice of atonement leads us to see more and more clearly whatever greed, aversion, and delusive certainty contributed to the harm we have caused. All this functions to serve our intimacy by lowering the barrier between ourselves and others. Humility, as opposed to shame, serves the cause of nonseparation by helping us to make deep contact with how thoroughly interdependent we are with our partner and with the world. Through the practice of atonement, we become gentler and more caring because we come to feel so deeply the pain and joy of others. The right hand is careful with the left hand because they are both part of the same whole.

We nurture intimacy with our partner through meeting their hurt and vulnerability and taking up the responsibility for caring for and not being separate from their vulnerability. We atone by sharing our vulnerability and fallibility, owning our capacity for harmfulness and our need for acceptance and grace. We move forward by asking to be forgiven and forgiving. We foster intimacy in each of these painfully counterintuitive, loving actions.

We atone by sharing our vulnerability and fallibility, owning our capacity for harmfulness and our need for acceptance and grace.

Forgiveness

For reconciliation to occur, repair or atonement must eventually be met with the practice of forgiveness. In the forgiveness literature, getting stuck in the flight-or-fight reaction after our partner has hurt us is referred to as suffering *unforgiveness*. The fight aspects of unforgiveness live in our desire for retribution, punishment, and retributive justice. Clinging to the powerful eye-for-an-eye desire for revenge has been shown to be corrosive to our own health and well-being. It is very much like drinking poison in the hope that the other person will die. The flight aspect of unforgiveness lives in our active avoidance of and turning away from our partner. We instinctively pull back and turn a cold shoulder toward the other as a way of protecting ourselves, and when we get stuck in that stance, we add to our own harm by clinging to active avoidance.

In the study of forgiveness, there are many circumstances under which reconciliation is dangerous or simply unavailable. Sometimes the people who caused harm remain harmful. Sometimes the people who caused harm are gone or unreachable for reconciliation, through either death or distance. However, the unavailability of reconciliation does not mean that the positive work of forgiveness cannot occur. We have learned that letting go of unforgiveness can be enough to free us from the trap that binds us and the poison that weakens us. When we are called to the practice of forgiveness in our intimate relationship, reconciliation is often the ultimate goal, but it does not have to be.

We often think about forgiveness as something that we must conjure up or build or create or lift in some way, as though we have to almost physically create forgiveness and are then stuck or failing in our willingness or capacity if we cannot muster forgiveness as an act of willpower. The language of letting go, however, points more directly at the actual manifestation of forgiveness as an invitation toward ease and a settling into our fundamental connectedness.

The actual manifestation of forgiveness is an invitation toward ease and a settling into our fundamental connectedness.

Intention, Attention, and Action with Forgiveness

I consider forgiveness a spiritual practice, because we move from protecting our ego to practicing compassion, because we heal the rift of separation to nurture heartfelt intimacy. When we are hurt, our ego often solidifies and becomes rigid, our view narrows exclusively to self-concern, and we constrict and separate. To actively move toward forgiveness and healing requires us to lower our ego barriers, to risk vulnerability, to heal the gap of separateness, and to prioritize intimacy over retribution and self-protective constriction.

How do we engage the practice of forgiveness in the service of our broader practice of intimacy? As with so much of intimacy practice, we start by setting our intention to forgive. We acknowledge that forgiving someone is not instantaneous, like flipping a light switch. Forgiveness is a journey that can both take a long time and traverse a lot of unforeseen and complicated terrain. We cannot simply will ourselves to the destination. We must travel there, step by step, until one day we break into the clearing and finally arrive.

And yet, though we cannot, through simple willpower, arrive instantaneously at forgiveness, we can very deliberately set ourselves out on the journey. We can deliberately take the first step toward forgiveness by simply stating our intention to do so—for example, "I haven't forgiven you yet, but I want to. I want to forgive you, and it is my intention to find my way there, with you, together."

Having set our intention, we turn our attention to how we might be embodying unforgiveness. When we sit down to meditate on forgiveness, we allow ourselves to receive, to touch deeply, all the ways that we are turning away from our partner and from our experience of vulnerability. Where might we be carrying unforgiveness in our body? As we breathe in and out, we feel the tension and the constriction of wanting retribution, the clinging of self-righteous umbrage, the weight of rage and anger protecting our underlying vulnerability. Feel the body turning away and wanting to escape, disappear, and flee from the complexity of continued connection.

We bring our full attention to each of the places where we are carrying unforgiveness, just allowing ourselves to feel them deeply and thoroughly. We might notice and even name our thoughts without acting on or nurturing them. As we become more intimate with the physical and mental experience, the constriction and fantasy of unforgiveness, we begin to loosen their hold on us. Perhaps we notice that they are not actually protecting us but only constraining and poisoning us. We practice allowing them to come and go without clinging to them for succor or safety. Perhaps we glimpse moments of freedom from unforgiveness and the lightness and healing that arise in its absence. We touch, if only briefly, the release and healing that is forgiveness as the absence of tension, fear, and anger. We don't reach for these experiences as a goal to be achieved so much as we open ourselves to being visited by them as we sit in communion with our bodies and minds just as they are in this moment.

The Steps to Practicing Forgiveness

How might we summarize the steps in the practice of forgiveness?

1. *Notice your reaction.* First, notice the maelstrom that is your fight-or-flight response. Pay attention to how this automatic hardwired physiological and psychological reaction solidifies into unforgiveness and the hardening of your ego barriers.
2. *Come to the cushion.* Next, sit still and upright in the heart of the storm, meeting it all with mindfulness and loving care. Touch into the vulnerability at the heart of your pain, and hold that vulnerability with tenderness and wisdom.
3. *Set an intention.* Then set your intention to let go of unforgiveness and to set foot on the path toward forgiveness. Vow to practice intimacy.
4. *Practice loving-kindness.* Bring an image of your partner to mind, or look at their picture with kind eyes and an open heart. Say to yourself or out loud, "May you be well. May you be free from harm. May you feel loved. May you be happy." Repeat this loving-kindness mantra every day. When you wake up. Before you greet your partner in the morning. Before you call or text them during the day. Before you close your eyes to sleep. I encourage you to notice how this practice affects your own heart and mind.
5. *Practice deep looking.* When you are fussy and unforgiving, you might not notice that you don't really look at your partner. You might glance or glare but no longer make loving eye contact or gaze deeply at their face. Looking deeply at your partner, looking them kindly in the eyes, opens an intimacy channel and softens the heart. If you have stopped looking at your partner, start again. See them for the beautiful, soft, fallible being that they are. Touch their vulnerability with your eyes.

Having planted the seeds of connection, we water them every day and sit patiently and faithfully awaiting their emergence. For ourselves, for each other, and for all beings.

The Heart of the Matter

In our relationships, we will cause and receive harm, whether great or small, every day and over and over again from this day forward and for the rest of our lives. We are but poor porcupines, longing for love and connection amidst an overabundance of quills and soft bellies. Intimacy requires our vulnerability and the vulnerability of others. And we must care for that vulnerability with unrelenting attention, love, and compassion. We must take up the practice of repair, atonement, and forgiveness as though our very lives depend on it.

Because they do.

Mindful Mantra

May you be well. May you be free from harm. May you be happy. May you be loved.

May I attend and tend to every harm that I will cause—both great and small.

May I respond to the hurts that I receive with grace and forgiveness.

May intimacy heal me, and you, and the world entire.

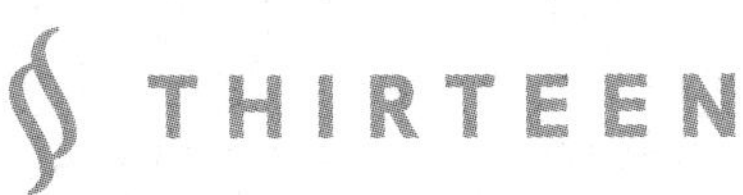

Facing Impermanence

INTIMACY WITH AGING, ILLNESS, AND DEATH

If you are coming to this chapter out of necessity, then let me first say that my heart is with your heart. You are in the midst of great change and likely experiencing pain, grief, confusion, and heartache. May you encounter this moment deeply. May you turn toward the path of intimacy as it unfolds before you. May you find wisdom for yourself and for all beings on this path.

In this chapter, we are heading into difficult, existential territory. Before we start, let's take a deep breath together, settling into this moment. Invite yourself to notice where you are and what you can see in your surroundings. Maybe notice what you can see outside your window—the breeze in the trees, the color of the sky. Notice any sounds you can hear—the whir and gurgle of the space that you are in. Bring your attention into your body. Do a quick scan of your physical experience and notice the sensations in the muscles of your arms, chest, back, shoulders, legs, feet, hands, and face. Take another deep breath and let some of the tension go with the outbreath. You are alive. Breathing in and breathing out. For now, this is enough. For now, this is everything.

In this chapter, we turn toward the great existential issues at the heart of long-term intimate relationships—aging, ill health, and death. When we weave our lives together with another person, we include everything. We include all the aspects of what it means to be a human being. We practice intimacy to know in our bones the truth of our interdependence—that whatever we are going through, our partner is also going through inseparably with us. If we are sick, then they are sick. If we are growing old, then they are growing old. If we are suffering, then they are suffering. If we are dying, then they are dying. For better or for worse. In sickness and in health. For richer or for poorer. To love and cherish. Until in death do we each part from this realm.

The Five Remembrances

In the communities in which I practice Zen meditation, at the start of almost all practice sessions, we recite together a small handful of readings, which almost always includes one called the Five Remembrances. The Five Remembrances is a statement of five truths. The mantra often strikes people new to them as rather surprisingly frank about life's existential issues but also just as often becomes one of their favorite recitations. In the practice, everyone who is gathered to meditate recites several chants together. In the case of the Five Remembrances, I often think we do this together as a way of holding each other through a shared recognition of our common humanity. We encourage ourselves and each other to reflect on these existential truths. We support each other in turning toward some of the most challenging aspects of our lives. I believe these are the places at which we are most likely to turn away from intimacy and thus perpetuate our experience of separateness and suffering. It is scary to turn toward our vulnerability to illness, old age, and death. So we need each other's help, support, encouragement, and compassion.

And, so, here it is, the Five Remembrances:

I am of the nature to grow old; there is no way to escape growing old.

I am of the nature to have ill health; there is no way to escape having ill health.

I am of the nature to die; there is no way to escape death.

All that is dear to me and everyone I love are of the nature of change; there is no way to escape being separated from them.

My deeds are my closest companions. I am born of my deeds; and I am their heir. My deeds are the ground on which I stand.

If you like, you are invited to recite this passage three times. Each time, as much as you can, I invite you to deeply feel the truth of each sentence in your bones, without turning away. This is existential exposure therapy and deep intimacy practice.

From our perspective in this book, I am inviting us all to take up each of these issues from the viewpoint of how we live them out in intimate relationship. In this chapter, we address the first three.

I Am of the Nature to Grow Old

We are of the nature to grow old; there is no way to escape growing old. And, if we are partnered, and lucky, we will grow old together.

The research literature reveals that relationship satisfaction commonly increases as we grow older. Most likely because the older we get, on average, the more life teaches us about acceptance and compassion. If a spiritual practice plays rough with the ego, then aging together is undoubtedly a spiritual practice. . . . if we let it be so. Aging together as a spiritual mindfulness practice involves turning toward intimacy with ongoing change.

Our bodies will change and keep changing. What we can and cannot do will continue to change. What we do with our time will change. Our perspective will change. Our families will change. Our responsibilities and social positions will change. And as each of these aspects of our lives change, our relationship will change right along with them. As our bodies grow into older bodies, we will be confronted again and again with the practice of letting go of our attachment to our and our partner's former appearance and abilities and acceptance of and curiosity about these new bodies that we have today.

Rather than suffer the loss of looking backward (though that is inescapably part of the wholeness of the experience), we might be invited to turn toward these bodies that we are blessed with today with love and curiosity. What can we experience with this body today? What can our beloved experience with their body today? Thus, rather than focus on what we can't do, we can focus on what we are capable of. Let's take these bodies out for a drive and see what they can do.

Intention, Attention, and Action with Growing Old Together

So at the beginning we set the intention to be fully and mindfully present in each unfolding moment of our aging together. We vow not to turn away but instead to embrace the flow of change as it unfolds for us and our beloved. We also vow to meet our wish that it were otherwise with the same wise compassion. Of course, we will have our moments when we will grumble about growing older and long for our younger selves. And, again, the invitation is to remember that our vow is to be as vividly awake in this moment, at this age, with this treasured other, as we can. We can say, "My love, as you grow older, I vow to see you with fresh eyes every day, to see you for the miraculous being that you are today, knowing that today is a precious gift that must be savored or lost."

Aging is just another word for change. As each moment accumulates into each day, each week, and each year, we are transformed together into something new. Our task is to bring attention to the transformation in each moment. You might wonder, *Are we getting older or newer? What is new about you and me today? What is here that wasn't here before? What is gone that used to be here?* The landscape of our lives and love is constantly shifting, and I invite us to treasure its newness with our attention. Bring gentle curiosity to just exactly what is new and here in this moment, without judgment, for us and our partner. It might go something like, "Huh? These pants don't fit. *That's* new! Where's our pile to donate to Goodwill?" "You've got a white hair in your eyebrow. *That's* new! Do you want to keep it, or shall I pluck it for you?"

New wrinkles, new knowledge, new perspectives, new aches, new abilities, new frailties, new fascinations, new annoyances—every day something new to notice and experience together—because we love each other, and we can. Eventually you might even notice that when you look deeply at just this unfolding moment, you don't find aging anywhere. The only thing here is just this. You don't feel "getting older." You only feel us.

The spiritual practice of aging together involves a lot of letting go. As life unfolds continually and relentlessly, we stay present to what is most vividly alive in this moment through the practice of letting go of the former moment, and letting go, and letting go. So we let go of who we were before so that we can appreciate who we are today. We let go of who our partner was yesterday, so that we can appreciate who they are today.

Rather than turning away from and fighting against that fact, we can embrace it as simply part of our particular and unique journey. We can savor what is today with fresh hands. Embrace with loving arms. To know you are my love made manifest and that today we are blessed. You might say to your partner, "I will not squander our time fretting about the future and regretting how our aging might unfold, but instead will hold you close today, speak to you with love and kindness today, keep you company and make you laugh today. Today I will love you like an all-consuming fire—with everything that I am. What a privilege to grow older with you."

I Am of the Nature to Have Ill Health

We all get sick from time to time. We will all suffer from periods in which we are significantly unwell, physically or mentally. As we age, it is not uncommon for ill health to become more and more a part of our day-to-day experience. The ills that we might suffer span the gamut from simple things like the common cold or a sprained ankle to significantly more challenging things like a cancer diagnosis or something chronic and progressive like dementia.

The main point here is that whatever we might be suffering from, our partner will also be suffering from. Whatever our struggle is individually, it is also being experienced simultaneously and relationally by our partner. When we catch a cold, our partner is also more likely to catch a cold. And even if they don't, we are going to be less available and less capable until we recover. We are also going to require more care.

The same holds true to an even greater extent if we develop something more serious, such as cancer. If we get a cancer diagnosis, so does our partner. We will each be scared, worried, and concerned, both for ourselves and for each other. As treatment diminishes our resources, it diminishes our partner's resources, too. We will encounter the realness of our mortality together, and each of us will respond to that threat in our own way. We will need their support and they will need ours.

My partner was diagnosed with breast cancer a few years before we started dating. She noticed a lump one morning while sitting up in bed, so small she could only just feel it, and more from the inside than from the outside. Wisely, she fought through her self-doubt and brought her fear and worry to her doctor. We are surrounded by the care of the compassionate. Her doctor helped her set in motion the long process of scans, biopsy, and diagnosis. At first the cancer was diagnosed as a type requiring an all-out, life-altering effort—surgery, chemotherapy, and radiation. She was terrified and heartbroken. First the surgery and then recovery. New wounds. New scars. Ancient fears. Then preparing for chemotherapy. New griefs and challenges. She cut her hair.

Showing up for chemotherapy defines the surreal. Sunny days. Friendly nurses. Coffee and snacks. And so many others here receiving the lifesaving poison. But she had a severe reaction to the chemotherapy drugs. Nurses leaping walls to get to her, to quell the anaphylaxis and put a brave face on a life-threatening moment. Then a whole-body cheetah rash that itched and bruised and meant harsher measures would be needed. While the doctors were debating the next course of action, she sought a second opinion from one of the leading oncologists in the country. They reanalyzed her biopsy and determined that the cancer was of a type that did not, in fact, require chemotherapy after all, and for which radiation treatment had a high likelihood of success.

Though she and I had been colleagues and friends before, we became closer throughout this frightening and difficult period of her life. In fact, in retrospect, it is clear that the very early seeds of our relationship were planted during this deeply existential period of ill health. We have since lived and loved into a relationship woven of strength and frailty, beautiful dreams, and genuine fears, vibrantly life affirming and just as vibrantly mortality affirming. We are together now, healthy and so very happy. And we live with a long-tailed shadow whispering *recurrence*. The truth of our interwovenness is palpable in every facet of our shared lives, including this one. The lingering threat of ill health, of cancer, is real, and we are, together, vigilant. Mindful of what is precious.

And ephemeral.

And perhaps this truth is at its most challenging when one of us is significantly unwell. When we are well, we are not separate. When we are unwell, we are not separate. When we are deeply aware of our interconnectedness and when we are coming forth from that place, we are engaged in the true practice of intimacy. We know ourselves and we know each other, and we are so much better able to act with love, compassion, and skill.

One of the most significant relational challenges that can arise when one partner is unwell is falling into a pattern in which one partner gets lost in the role of the caretaker and the other gets lost in the role of the one who is taken care of (see Chapter 3). Of course, at first it makes sense that the attachment system is activated when one partner is sick. We are each other's attachment figures, and when one of is rattled, upset, or ungrounded by life, we very naturally seek out our partner for support, solace, and encouragement. That is how attachment systems work, both between partners and between children and their caregivers.

Intention, Attention, and Action with Ill Health

How do we practice with moments of ill health (and the threat of ill health) in ourselves, in our partner, and in our relationship? As with all opportunities for mindfulness practice (and *all moments* are opportunities for mindfulness practice), we begin by orienting ourselves toward our intention, the intention of intimacy. Intimacy means nonseparation, wholeness, and appreciation of the nondual nature that is our birthright. Thus intimacy involves turning toward what we are turning away from, allowing what we are disallowing, integrating what we are separating, and reweaving what we are tearing apart.

When we are the one who is unwell, how do we practice turning toward intimacy? By simply acknowledging to ourselves that we are sick. This might seem simple, but if we look deeply, we are likely to discover ways in which we try to deny that we are sick, or ways in which we engage in subtle forms of self-aggression because we are sick. We tough it out, so we can get our work done. We go to the meeting anyway, because we don't want to admit that we're sick, we want to be strong and reliable. We don't want to overreact, or we just don't want the inconvenience of being sick. Maybe we don't want to admit to ourselves that we might be contagious, so we just don't think about it and instead let the momentum of the day have the wheel. It can be hard to turn toward and simply admit to ourselves that we are sick.

When we are unwell, the simple self-compassionate act of admitting that we are unwell can be a tremendous source of relief. It releases us from the struggle of trying to suppress, deny, ignore, or simply soldier on—each of which takes genuine effort. We often don't even notice how much effort we are putting into trying to deny that we are sick until we stop and just let ourselves feel the way we feel. Ceasing the desperate act of separation is almost always a moment of real relief. It is important to name it: "I think I have a cold (or the flu or COVID)"; "My back is really hurting today"; "I am feeling a lot of anxiety"; "I'm suffering a lot of symptoms of depression today."

When it is our partner who is unwell, how do we practice turning toward intimacy? Again, simply acknowledging, accepting, and experiencing what is undeniably true. Our partner is sick. Whether it be cancer, depression, injury, or dementia, the first step is turning toward and welcoming the unwelcome. We might notice all the obvious and subtle ways that we turn away from, reject, and deny our partner's illness. It can be so hard to simply turn toward and acknowledge with a compassionately aching heart, "My love is sick. . . . and I am not medicine."

Indeed, one of the most challenging aspects of intimacy when our partner is unwell is the degree to which we are helpless in the face of it. We are not the medicine that will make them well. We are not the cure for their disease, nor do we have access to it. We can love them with our whole heart, and we can't fix them. This is hard, but it is the truth in this moment.

We may not be the medicine, but our presence matters. Our presence matters to them, and it matters to us. So we practice turning toward our partner. Turning toward their unwellness. Turning toward our desperate wish that it were otherwise. Turning toward stillness. And presence. Ceasing our desperate efforts of fight or flight in the face of a partner's illness and simply release into compassionate presence. All this so that we might bask in our interconnectedness and know that, as Rumi reminds us, *love is the whole thing.*

From Struggle to Serenity

Struggling with being sick makes us unskillful by limiting our access to the full array of what is simply true in the moment. For example, if we have the flu, and we are downplaying or otherwise denying it, then we are less likely to take proper care of ourselves and thus more likely to stay sick longer, or even get sicker. In turning away from or denying our interconnectedness, we are less likely to take proper care of others, and we simply go the meeting, party, or event anyway, thus running the risk of making our friends and colleagues sick and simply perpetuating the cycle of suffering.

When we acknowledge that we or our partner are unwell, we stop getting in the way of our own healing, and we stop blocking our access to wisdom and skillful action.

After acknowledging that we are sick, we may even share that we are sick or unwell as part of our intimacy practice. Sharing cultivates intimacy and understanding in our relationship with our partner and with others. When we pretend that we are fine or good, we hide our authentic self from others and block the path of intimacy. We have become so used to answering the question, "How are you?" with "Fine/good/great" that it can be genuinely shocking when someone answers honestly.

A former colleague had a habit of answering the hallway question "How are you?" as though the person were genuinely interested in his honest answer. As I passed him in the hall and greeted him with "How are you?" he would say "My stomach has been bothering me today" or "I'm feeling ready for a nap." At first being met with anything other than "fine" seemed like a break in social etiquette, but after a while, I noticed that I started to see him more clearly, appreciate seeing him in the hallways more joyfully, feel closer to him as a fellow human being. Can this be another component of your practice, to share your feelings, your pain, your fears, your vulnerabilities in the service of connection and closeness? Try it.

PRACTICING WITH ILLNESS: SIMULTANEOUS TRUTHS

When you stop struggling with being sick and simply acknowledge that, in addition to all the other things that are true about you today, you are also sick, then you are immediately more whole, more integrated, and more intimate. Because of that, you also have access to the full perspective needed to act with skill and wisdom. Acknowledging that you (or your partner) are sick is a spiritual practice because it promotes intimacy, because it is humbling and compassionate and acknowledges our interdependent nature. The key is sometimes just the difference between *but* and *and*. The word *and* allows that both things are simultaneously true and is thus more whole, integrated, and intimate. *But* separates and puts two experiences at odds with each other, which ultimately makes us less skillful, robs us of our innate wisdom, and causes more suffering.

Read the following statements and notice the different experience when using *but* versus *and*. Then pull out your journal and write your own *and* statements. Say them to yourself when you need a kind and loving reminder of how to be intimate in this moment.

- I am sick, *but* I have to attend this meeting. I can't afford to slow down.
- I am sick, *and* it's important to attend this meeting, and slowing down has consequences.
- My partner is sick, *but* I can't just stop getting my work done.
- My partner is sick, *and* there are so many things that must get done.
- I have many things I need to accomplish today, *but* I have physical therapy this afternoon.
- I have many things I need to accomplish today, *and* I am going to need more rest than usual because the physical therapy is exhausting.
- I am injured, *but* I'm supposed to go on a retreat with my friend who's having a hard time.
- I am injured, *and* I can still be a good friend and source of encouragement.
- My partner is unwell, *but* I need someone to lean on.
- My partner is unwell, *and* I can lean on them even while they lean on me.

In other words, we work with everything that is simultaneously true, so that we can behave as wisely as possible. We might cancel meetings that can be put off, reschedule them to video conferencing, or, if we do go physically to the meeting, we might wear a mask to protect our colleagues. When we turn toward intimacy and acknowledge that we are sick, we very naturally take better care of ourselves and each other.

The Gift of Needing Your Partner

Interestingly, it's also not uncommon in the couples that I work with for partners to deny to each other that they are unwell. In my experience, this is more common in men, who often tell me that they don't want to be a burden or add to their partner's problems. So often, as men, we are taught to suck it up and soldier on, that our ill health becomes a source of shame or embarrassment for us. This phenomenon isn't exclusive to men, by any stretch, just slightly more common.

Being unwell can be an enormous source of vulnerability, especially to the degree that we have been mocked or shamed for being weak or lazy, or if our role models prided themselves on soldiering on through sickness or injury. The sense of shame or embarrassment for being sick or injured is itself an important opportunity for practice. When we notice that we are hiding the fact that we are feeling unwell or in pain from our partner, we can use that moment of noticing to feel for the way in which it is making us feel vulnerable—vulnerable to being mocked, vulnerable to feeling like a burden, vulnerable to being seen as weak or incapable. For many of us, that vulnerability is so raw that being tended to with care and kindness actually makes us angry. We prefer to be ignored or even encouraged to soldier on because it makes us feel strong, admired, and capable. Too many of us have been rewarded for turning away from intimacy and shamed for admitting that we might need care.

But, in our intimate relationships, needing and asking for care is a gift. Trusting our partner with the vulnerability that we feel when we are sick, injured, or mentally or emotionally unwell is an act of entrustment. That act of turning toward when we need care acknowledges our love, trust, and faith in our partner. And, as partners, we long to be a source of trusted care for the people we love. We want to know that they can turn to us in a time of need and that we will care for them with love and skill. We long to feel competent and effective when our partner needs us.

As in all our intimacy practice, the practice is about turning toward what is undeniably true and makes us feel vulnerable. We are both vulnerable to our own ill health and simultaneously exquisitely vulnerable to our partner's ill health. Denying our vulnerability tears us in half, shuts us off from ourselves and each other, and makes us hard and lonely. Reminding ourselves that we are all vulnerable to illness, injury, and mental/emotional distress deepens our experience of our common humanity, softens our hearts, releases our compassion and mercy, and connects us back to ourselves and each other.

As we have discussed throughout this book, vulnerability is the gateway to intimacy. Vulnerability is openness to connection. Vulnerability is acknowledgment of our place in the universe. When we can acknowledge to ourselves that we are unwell, we are at greater peace and better able to care for ourselves with skill and wisdom. When we can share with our partner that we are unwell, we create opportunities for care and the receiving of care, embodying that we are each other's attachment figures, and strengthening our intimate connection. When we can acknowledge that our partner is unwell and that because they are suffering, we are suffering, then we can access fathomless compassion and skillful care for both of us. We will row this leaky boat together, for ourselves, for each other, and for all beings.

And, even when we are unwell, we can still provide care, love, and connection to others. This continues the practice of both–and. You can say, "I am sick and I am still capable of care and kindness. I am mentally/emotionally distressed, and I can still be of service and a source of loving connection." Similarly, when your partner is unwell, you can still need and reach out for care and connection. You can cry on their shoulder, even while you are bringing their medicine. We are us, and this is thus, and so we shall be for always.

We are of the nature to have ill health; there is no way to escape having ill health.

PRACTICING MINDFUL AWARENESS OF ILLNESS WITH OUR PARTNER

You can begin practicing with illness in your relationship by settling down on your seats together, breathing deeply together, and letting it out slowly.

1. Focus your attention on your breath as it comes in and goes out, wherever it is most palpable to you in the moment.
2. Feel your partner's presence next to you, also breathing, and looking deeply.
3. Having anchored your present-moment attention in the flow of your breath, turn your attention to where in your body you are feeling unwell or where you might be feeling your connection to your partner's suffering. Scan your body from head to foot, slowly feeling your way into each section of your body. Notice areas where there are aches and pains. Maybe a small sharp pain in the upper left quadrant of your right eye socket. Maybe your shoulders are achy, heavy, or tired. Maybe your head is stuffy, and it is hard to breathe out of your nose. Maybe you feel the buzz and tension of anxiety.
4. As you bathe each area of your body in loving attention, feel each sensation deeply and with curiosity. Welcome and accept all the sensations

arising in the moment. Acknowledge to yourself: *I am feeling unwell* or *I am feeling my connectedness to my partner, who is unwell.*

5. Discover that there are areas of your body that do not feel unwell, sad, worried, or anxious. There are areas that feel fine, relaxed, and healthy. Also notice that areas that feel unwell or anxious are made of an array of different sensations that arise and fall away, that flow and pulse, that undulate and change.
6. Simply acknowledge that this is what it feels like right now to be unwell or worried. Meet it and honor it by allowing yourself some rest and ease. Or soothing medicine. Or go for a refreshing walk. Or reach out to friends.
7. Listen closely to your intimate experience, discovering with compassion and curiosity how best to care for each other—your bodies and minds. This is love.

I Am of the Nature to Die

To be separated by death is the nature of lasting intimacy. There is a quote by Ram Dass that speaks quite beautifully to this aspect of our nature. He writes, "We are all just walking each other home." I find this such a beautiful sentiment and gentle reminder. Whenever I am feeling fussy with someone, my partner, a family member, a student, or colleague, if I am lucky enough to remember that we are all just walking each other home, then I am transformed. And this is, for me, the spiritual gift of turning toward intimacy with our shared mortality—that we are both on this short journey together.

When I remember that we are just walking each other home, I am gentled, my heart softens, I become compassion. Compassion for whoever I am with and compassion for myself. I don't have to do anything else. I don't have to say anything about it or impose my view on the other person. I just keep it to myself. But I move differently. I see with kinder eyes. I speak with more love and tenderness. Perhaps, if I'm lucky, I am guided by greater wisdom.

The invitation to not turn away from an enduring awareness of our shared mortality is one of the most significant aspects of a thoroughgoing intimacy practice. There can be no wholeness, no true intimacy, no genuine union if we remain defended against, turned away, and separate from this most existential of truths. All spiritual traditions attempt to help us integrate this fundamental aspect of our human experience. So, too, does much of psychology. In particular, existential/humanistic psychology posits that what they call *death anxiety* is at the heart of much of our anxiety and suffering.

And, as difficult as it is to mindfully turn toward and integrate our own mortality, it is even harder to do so for the people we hold most dear. We are so strongly motivated by even the thought of what the pain of that loss might be that we deny and turn away from acknowledging and honoring our shared mortality. That is precisely why regular mindfulness practices like the Five Remembrances were created by our wise ancestors to turn us toward, with an abundance of compassion, what we would otherwise continually turn away from. If intimacy is our salvation, we cannot separate illness, aging, and death from the whole. Our mortality is an inextricable part of us. Our beloved's mortality is an inextricable part of them. And to love them intimately, we must not turn away from that truth.

In a spiritual practice of intimacy, awareness of both our vitality and our mortality is an essential part of our ongoing mindfulness practice. Awareness of both our resilience and our fragility is acknowledgment of the whole. We are not separate, by even a hair's breadth. The Buddhist scripture Dhammapada reminds us that "unlike those who don't realize we're here on the verge of perishing, those who do: their quarrels are stilled." The gift of wholeness in this mindfulness practice is a much more effortless peace. But to achieve that peace, we must first know our ephemerality.

My older sister was diagnosed with fourth-stage breast cancer when she was 32. I remember vividly the day she called me to tell me. I was in my apartment in Seattle in the sixth year of my doctoral program. I can recall the dismal brown of the kitchen cabinets that I was staring at as she cried on the phone—heartbroken and terrified. My sister had always been such a source of strength and joy in my life. Her terror was my terror. Her heartbreak was my heartbreak. Over the course of the next four years, we all lived with the most painful awareness of how close death was to her and thus to all of us. It is perhaps cliché, but cliché for a reason, that during those years, we were closer and more authentic with each other than ever before. We were all living much more vividly the gratitude for life and fear of death that mix our daily ration.

My father, for my whole life, had always been a reactively irritable man. In retrospect, I have come to realize that it was rooted in clinical levels of anxiety and deeply ingrained shame. But, nevertheless, the lived experience was traversing the minefield of his hair-trigger anger. I was always tense in his presence and relieved in his absence. When my sister died, it broke him. Honestly, it broke all of us. But for my dad, in particular, grief shook him to the core, unmoored him, blew apart the fragile walls that he had built to protect himself, laid his heart bare, naked, and defenseless. And, as it does for all of us, his grief transformed him. Within the following years he became gentle, empathic, protective, and generous in ways that I had never seen before. His sharp edges blasted off; he became a hugger and a baby snuggler. Easily moved to tears, he ended all phone calls with an "I love you" that, honestly, I didn't even know he knew how to say before. He gardened. He gave his time. He could still get fussy, but that part of him became minuscule in comparison.

I can't say any of us ever really recovered. We all still miss my sister terribly to this day. But until creeping dementia stole him away, the heart that grief uncovered for my dad was a treasure. Intimate, intimate.

I share this story to highlight that a relational intimacy practice that embraces our fragility completes our intimacy. Well, "completes" might imply too much. Intimacy is a living experience that breathes and flows endlessly. But we cannot approach the true depths of it without mending the gap that separates us from our shared mortality. We are of the nature to die. There is no way to escape death.

Intention, Attention, and Action with Death

How do we practice intimacy with our impermanent nature?

Whether this is a moment in which death is close at hand for one of us, or one in which we are simply acknowledging our shared mortality, the key practice, as always, is turning toward, loving attention, and stillness.

PRACTICING INTIMACY WITH OUR MORTALITY

1. Situate your body so you can be still and upright for a few minutes. Maybe 10 minutes. Maybe 25. Sit next to your partner. Or perhaps simply bring your partner to mind and to heart. Embrace their presence. Let yourself feel their presence in your whole being.
2. Bring your attention to your breath and your body. Take a deep breath,

and let it out slowly. Breathe their presence in. Practice your present-centeredness for a few breaths.

3. Allow yourself to feel your partner's presence and the quality of that presence. Notice how the experience fluxes and flows, constantly changing and endlessly arising—ephemeral and vivid.
4. Notice how in this moment your lived experience of your partner simultaneously consists of arriving and falling away. Coming and going. Life and death. In equal measure, ceaseless and ungraspable. This ungraspability and ceaseless arising is the true nature of the living moment. This is the lived experience of our fundamental impermanence. As we stand in the river, is it arriving or is it departing? As we stand in this moment of our shared lives, are we coming into being or are we dissipating? Life and death as separate from each other perhaps makes less and less sense. There is just this flow. Just this thusness. You are just walking together. You are just walking each other home.

If our partner is dying, we can sit with them. Keep them company. Touch them. Bring them gifts. Tell them stories. Make them laugh. Live this moment with them like an all-consuming fire. Fully present. With nothing held back. Bring them comfort. Soothe their fears. Walk each other home.

If our partner has passed away, continuing their transformation into new aspects of the universe, we can grieve for them. Let grief be our guide into deeper intimacy. Allow its ebb and flow. Let our heart break and beat and break and beat. There is a powerful invitation in bringing our grief to formal meditation practice. To allow ourselves to be with the great ocean of grief in stillness.

Even from our deathbed, we can turn toward intimacy with our partner. Though we may be slipping away, we can still pat our partner's hand and offer comfort and love. We can still be fully present and vividly alive—right up to the point where we can't. And even then, who knows?

But none of these precious moments of intimacy can be available to us if we turn away from these most challenging bits of being human. If we deny our impermanence, if we turn away from our mortality, then we necessarily turn away from our partner and from life. One cannot embrace life in half measures. We either step forward fully or we hang back. There is no in between. It is only by embracing our common humanity, our shared vulnerability, that we are offered entry into true intimacy.

The Heart of the Matter

Intimacy with our lives, just the way they are, is the gift of contemplative practice. The Five Remembrances call us to turn toward the deepest, most existential aspects of our lives together in our intimate relationships. Right here, in the heart of aging, illness, death, change, and interconnectedness, we can practice continually and repeatedly turning toward each other, holding each other close, comforting and celebrating our shared fate—and, hand in hand, walking each other home.

Mindful Mantra

You, my beloved, and I are of the nature to grow old. May we age beautifully and courageously together.

You, my beloved, and I are of the nature to have ill health. May we care tenderly for ourselves and each other whenever either of us is sick.

You, my beloved, and I are of the nature to die. May we live every second turned toward each other and our shared life, savoring the moment and sucking the marrow—tumbling through the free fall together.

Forever and ever.

Amen.

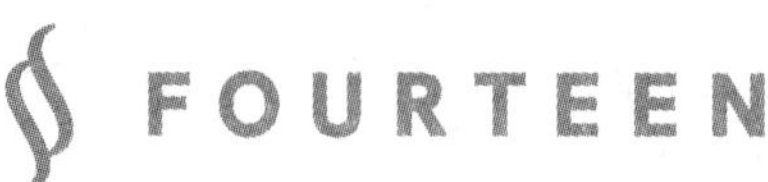

FOURTEEN

Walking the Intimate Path

THE WHOLE WORLD IS MEDICINE

In the 87th koan of the Blue Cliff Record (a collection of Zen Buddhist koans), the teacher, Yunmen, says to his students, "Medicine and illness correspond to each other. The whole world is medicine. Who are you?"

Medicine and illness write love letters to each other. The whole universe is medicine. What about you?

What about you?

Where in the eyes of your beloved is the medicine that you've been seeking your whole life? Where in the indecipherable text message? Where in the erotic touch? The frustrated sigh? The fumbled compliment? The poorly worded critique? The declaration of undying love? The complaint about the unloaded dishwasher? The panicked trip to the emergency room? The broken jar of spaghetti sauce? The unfolded laundry? The soft kiss? The held hand? The disappointment? The hurt? The joy? The encouragement? All the highs and lows and in-betweens?

The whole world is medicine for the illness of separation—deep in your heart, deep in your partner's heart. In the places where you are most vulnerable, and your partner is most tender. Everything that arises, in every moment of our lives, can be a source of healing. Everything that arises, in every moment of our lives, can be a cure to our loneliness. Everything that arises, in every moment of our lives, can be the balm for our deepest heartache, a teacher of our interconnectedness, a gateway to the path of true intimacy.

Everything that we are seeking in our search for awakening, enlightenment, wholeness, connection. . . . intimacy, is to be found, every day and in every moment, right here in our closest relationship. Mindful awareness of each vibrantly passing moment between you and your beloved is vividly demonstrating and enacting all the qualities of boundless connection.

It is said that the awakened ones teach only the cure to our suffering: the suffering that arises from our conviction that we are separate and alone, bereft and endangered, forever doomed to struggle against the tide of distress, dread, and disappointment.

In this place, the whole world is medicine.

May you and your beloved be well.
May you be free from harm.
May you both feel loved.
May you both be happy.
May you and your beloved bless the world with your love
And show us all the way.

The Heart of the Heart of the Matter

Right now, as you read this, that longing in your heart is the longing for true intimacy. Right now, as you read this, you are the intimacy that you seek. Right now, as you read this, you and your beloved, together, are the fulfillment of your endless seeking. With great energy and sincerity, contemplate this arising moment deeply. Practice mindfulness of this ceaselessly emerging moment while sitting together, walking together, and lying down together. Have faith that intimacy is your shared birthright.

Engage every moment of your relationship as a spiritual practice. Turn toward everything that is most deeply true about what it is like to be these two precious human beings together. Welcome all the joy and heartache with equal grace. Embrace both the quills and the warm soft bodies of our shared nature. Practice diligently when you sit down in formal meditation. Practice lovingly when you engage your world together. We suffer from the illness of imagined separation—and the whole universe is medicine. May you drink deeply each drop together. May the intimacy you seek find you right where you are—together, holding hands, walking each other home.

Index

About the Author

James V. Cordova, PhD, is Distinguished Professor of Psychology at Clark University. A leader in relationship research and couple therapy, he is the developer of the Marriage Checkup, an innovative approach to improving relationship health. Dr. Cordova is a longtime teacher of Zen meditation who is passionate about enriching couples' connections through both psychological insights and mindfulness. He divides his time between Worcester, Massachusetts, and Santa Fe, New Mexico.